T0315329

Vaccines: Truth, Lies, and Controversy

Peter C. Gøtzsche, DrMedSci

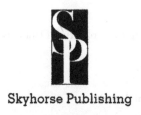

Skyhorse Publishing

Skyhorse Publishing books may be purchased in bulk at special discounts for sales promotion, corporate gifts, fund-raising, or educational purposes. Special editions can also be created to specifications. For details, contact the Special Sales Department, Skyhorse Publishing, 307 West 36th Street, 11th Floor, New York, NY 10018 or info@skyhorsepublishing.com.

Skyhorse® and Skyhorse Publishing® are registered trademarks of Skyhorse Publishing, Inc.®, a Delaware corporation.

Visit our website at www.skyhorsepublishing.com.

10 9 8 7 6 5 4 3 2

Library of Congress Cataloging-in-Publication Data is available on file.

Print ISBN: 978-1-5107-6219-0

Printed in the United States of America

Contents

Acknowledgments

I am very grateful for the information I have received from many researchers and patient advocates, including Alberto Donzelli and Manuel Martínez-Lavín. I wish to thank especially Peter Aaby, who is an astute observer who reports what he sees, unconstrained by prevailing paradigms and guidelines, and sometimes with great personal costs; and Rebecca Chandler for a critical reading of the manuscript.

Abbreviations

CDC: Centers for Disease Control and Prevention
EMA: European Medicines Agency
FDA: Food and Drug Administration
MMR: measles, mumps and rubella
WHO: World Health Organization

1

The Many Conflicting Messages about Vaccines

This book will help you navigate in the bewildering, and often contradictory, flood of information about vaccines. The information I provide is not a replacement for consultations with healthcare professionals but might empower you to engage in meaningful and informed discussions. You might also decide to make your own decisions. The conclusions I draw after having studied the evidence are personal; other researchers might arrive at different conclusions, as an element of judgment will always be involved.

Some vaccinations are so beneficial that we should all get them, while others should not be used except for special circumstances. Some are so controversial that many healthcare professionals do not use them for themselves even though they are officially recommended, e.g., influenza vaccines.

We must evaluate carefully each vaccine, one by one, assessing the balance between its benefits and harms, just as we do for other drugs, and then form an opinion about whether we think the vaccine is worth getting or recommending to other people.

The key issues are these: What is the risk of getting infected by the bacterium or virus the vaccine is directed against, and what is the risk of getting seriously harmed or dying because of the infection? What is the chance of avoiding an infection by vaccination, and what is the risk of getting seriously harmed or dying because of the vaccination?

As for other preventive measures, it can be difficult to provide evidence-based advice about vaccinations that apply universally because disease prevalence is important for decision making. All drugs have harms, and if your risk of contracting an infection is very low, it might not be worthwhile to run the risk of getting seriously harmed by the vaccine, even if this risk is also very low. In other cases, the benefits of a vaccine are so obvious compared to its harms that very few people should not get vaccinated, like those who suffer from severe immune deficiency and a live attenuated vaccine is being used, or those who are allergic to some of the vaccine's constituents.

This is straightforward and uncontroversial, but one reason why vaccines may confuse people is that they have become a battlefield. There are fundamentalists on both sides of the debate who ignore the evidence or manipulate it to further their agendas. When people who think the end justifies the means work for governmental or international agencies, the official advice about vaccines can become misleading, and the consequences can be serious. Citizens might decide to reject all vaccines when they find out they have been fooled by the authorities in relation to a particular one where they were already in doubt. I shall give many examples in this book that prove we cannot always trust official recommendations about vaccines, or the way authorities interpret the evidence.

The fundamentalists on the other side also cause harm. The worst of them reject all vaccines as a matter of "principle," and they have considerable influence via social media. It is unwise and unscientific to be universally against vaccines. It is like being against all drugs or all people. Some are good, some are bad, but if we reject all our fellow human beings, we will have no life, and if we reject all drugs, including badly needed blood transfusions, we might die.

The hard-core people even reject the measles vaccine, although it has saved millions of lives and still does (see next chapter). Their "back-to-nature" romanticism that it should somehow be better to let our children suffer from measles rather than avoiding measles through vaccination is misguided and will lead to numerous deaths and cases of severe brain damage. For measles, and other highly contagious infections, herd immunity is important. To prevent measles epidemics, vaccinating about 95% of the population is necessary, and we therefore have a joint societal responsibility toward one another to ensure that we get vaccinated. If you disagree, you should not throw my book away but read at least the next chapter. It will likely change your mind.

People who reject all vaccines and are totally resistant to rational arguments and findings from high-quality science going against their beliefs are often called anti-vaxxers. I do not like calling people anti-something. People who criticize the huge consumption of psychiatric drugs for valid scientific reasons are often called anti-psychiatry by psychiatrists, which they are not;

they are pro-people. I prefer to use the term "vaccine deniers," since they deny the science, just as there are Holocaust deniers and people who deny that man ever set foot on the Moon. The other camp I shall call "vaccine advocates," even though this term is too kind for those of them who are as unreasonable as the vaccine deniers when they say we should accept all vaccines without asking questions.

The rhetoric is sharp, not only from vaccine deniers, but also from vaccine advocates. For example, the British Health Minister has said that "Those people who campaign against vaccination are campaigning against science. The science is settled. . . . Those who have promoted the anti-vaccination myth are morally reprehensible, deeply irresponsible and have blood on their hands."[1]

Debates about vaccines are often so polarized that sensible discussion is impossible. As soon as legitimate questions are raised, the pro-vaccine camp may cry "anti-vaxxer" or ask if you are for or against vaccines.

Unfortunately, vaccine deniers are so powerful in the United States that it has led to self-censorship for truth-seeking scientists. A *New York Times* reporter wrote:

> When I tried to report on unexpected or controversial aspects of vaccine efficacy or safety, scientists often didn't want to talk with me. When I did get them on the phone, a worrying theme emerged: Scientists are so terrified of the public's vaccine hesitancy that they are censoring themselves, playing down undesirable findings and perhaps even avoiding undertaking studies that could show unwanted effects. Those who break these unwritten rules are criticized. The goal is to protect the public—to ensure that more people embrace vaccines—but in the long-term, the approach will backfire. Our arsenal of vaccines is exceptional, but it could always be better. Progress requires scientific candor and a willingness to ask inconvenient questions.[2]

A researcher, who published a paper showing that the flu vaccine was not particularly effective in the elderly, was no longer invited to meetings. Another researcher and her Canadian colleagues found data suggesting that flu vaccination might increase the risk of infection with other flu strains. They replicated their findings in five different studies and then shared the data with trusted colleagues: "There was tremendous pushback and some questioned whether the findings were appropriate for publication."[3] But their results were published.[4]

There is no doubt that stifling scientific inquiry is far more dangerous than publishing freely, and it leads to cherry-picking data, which is exactly what the vaccine deniers do: "Vaccines can't be refined if researchers ignore inconvenient data. Moreover, vaccine scientists will earn a lot more public trust, and overcome a lot more unfounded fear, if they choose transparency over censorship."[5]

We should try to understand where the vaccine denial comes from. Parents of children with developmental disorders like autism are seeking an explanation. It is not surprising that they may question the safety of a vaccine received shortly before the symptoms appeared, and it is not appropriate to label them anti-vaxxers. It is not surprising either that there are thousands of such parents, as billions of children are vaccinated. Their sheer numbers do not prove anything. The hypothesis that the measles vaccine can cause autism has been convincingly refuted, and the research that gave rise to it has been shown to be fraudulent (see next chapter).

Consumer advocate Kim Witczak has compared the vaccine industry with the "depression pill industry" and has described her experiences with name-calling.[6] She went into advocacy on drug safety as a result of malpractice: her husband was prescribed a depression pill for insomnia and the horrific harms he experienced drove him into suicide.[7] Both industries and their paid allies among doctors attack anyone who criticizes their drugs. If you argue, based on the best science you could find, that depression pills don't seem to work but drive some people, both children and adults, into suicide or violence, you are called "anti-psychiatry" by professors of psychiatry who protect their guild interests. I have experienced this several times from professors who have no valid counterarguments.[8]

Witczak has been called a Scientologist on multiple occasions, including when she was invited by the late Senator Ted Kennedy to testify before the US Senate about ways to improve the FDA and postmarket surveillance of drugs.[9] When she collected her bags afterward, a senator told her that the national lobbyist for the *National Alliance for the Mentally Ill*, which calls itself a "grassroots organization," stopped by all the senators' offices and told them not to believe a word she had said in the hearing because she was a Scientologist. This national alliance is so heavily supported by drug industry money—$12 million between 1996 and 1999—that it is fair to consider it corrupt.[10]

There are good reasons why people can become skeptical toward vaccines in general, or at least ask questions about them. The business practice of drug companies involves organized crime where cheating with the clinical trials and in marketing is common and has led to hundreds of thousands of deaths.[11] It is also clear that we cannot trust our drug regulators, who allow far too many dangerous drugs on to the market and are very slow to take them off again when the evidence for their lethal effects accumulates.[12]

It does not further public trust that official advice about vaccines, e.g., from national boards of health or from WHO, are derived from the results of industry-funded trials and from statements by drug regulators, or that many of the people who participate in drug regulation or formulate advice and guidelines have financial conflicts of interest in relation to vaccine manufacturers.

Another reason for sound skepticism is that very few or none of the pivotal clinical trials of vaccines include an untreated control group. It is a requirement for registration of drugs that randomized trials have been carried out where one group received the drug and the control group received placebo or nothing. This allows assessment of both the benefits and the harms of drugs. I have done research on nonvaccine drugs for decades and was shocked when I learned through my work with vaccines against human papilloma virus (HPV) that the regulatory requirements are much less for vaccines. Almost all the HPV vaccine trials have a control group receiving a hepatitis vaccine or a strongly immunogenic adjuvant, which makes it impossible to find out what the harms of the HPV vaccines are (see Chapter 6).

A bad reason for skepticism is when people draw conclusions about a cause-effect relationship when someone falls ill after being vaccinated. Yet many people are quick at drawing conclusions where none can be drawn. A US vaccine denier wrote to me that she had a neighbor ten houses down the street that had given her two-year-old the MMR vaccine two weeks earlier, and now the kid had high fever, was screaming insistently, and had banged his head against the wall for a week. I replied: "The child you mention could simply have acquired an infection at the same time. These things happen." In fact, it is highly unlikely that the kid's disease was caused by the vaccine (see next chapter).

The vaccine denier also asked me if I had any data showing that the MMR was a safe vaccine. That is not a relevant question. No drugs are safe. If we want to use drugs, we'll need to accept that some people will be harmed. We use drugs that do more good than harm, and the MMR vaccine is surely in that category.

Finally, she drew my attention to page 43 in a 1978 prelicense study for the MMR vaccine submitted to the FDA that Del Bigtree, the producer of the film *Vaxxed* (see next chapter), has posted on his website.[13] She wrote:

"That study says the 54% of the children in test groups got very ill and they only followed the groups for 43 days." However, page 43 does not say that the toddlers "got very ill"; it noted that upper respiratory and gastro-intestinal infections were reported in about 55% and 40% of the vaccinees, respectively. Such percentages are not useful, as we do not know how many toddlers would have acquired such infections without having been vacci-nated. Perhaps there were epidemics of such infections in the institutions that cared for the toddlers. Furthermore, the parents gave informed consent and knew they should report any issues with their children, which is likely to lead to considerable overreporting.

The immune system is immensely complicated, and it is not possible to predict which nonspecific effects a targeted vaccine might have. Vaccines can affect nontargeted infectious diseases both positively and negatively. Danish professor Peter Aaby has done ground-breaking research in this area spanning 40 years.[14] His group has published many papers that provide sup-port to their hypothesis that live attenuated vaccines decrease total mortal-ity while nonlive vaccines increase total mortality. The measles vaccine, for example, decreases mortality much more than what can be explained by its effect on preventing measles. The sequence of vaccinations also seems to be important for total mortality, and it is best to end with a live vaccine. Such observations do not render decision making about vaccines easy.

Bacillus Calmette-Guérin (BCG) for tuberculosis and the measles vac-cine probably reduce mortality from pneumonia and sepsis. In contrast, the combined diphtheria, tetanus, and pertussis (DTP) vaccine is suspected to double overall mortality in low-income countries, which is worrying because the vaccine apparently induces tolerance and increases the risk of unrelated infections, in particular respiratory infections, which are bigger killers than the targeted diseases in such settings[15] (see more about this in Chapter 8). These findings did not make Aaby popular at WHO headquar-ters. Public health messages become difficult when such totally unexpected results appear and become supported by subsequent studies.

There are important differences between vaccines and other drugs. The effect of the vaccine can change. It may have been developed for strains of viruses or bacteria different from those that currently exist in the target population, and there may be genetic, epidemiological, demographic, or environmental differences affecting the target population that modify the efficacy of the vaccine.

My rule of thumb is that if a vaccine is part of the official vaccination program in some countries but not in others of similar standing, then it is not important to get yourself or your child vaccinated. An example is the rotavirus vaccine against diarrhea, which is not on the childhood vaccine program in Denmark even though we had a strong lobby group promoting it. Yet again, global recommendations cannot be made. In low-income countries where infant diarrhea is an important cause of death, vaccination against rotavirus can be a good idea (see Chapter 8).

* * *

You should know a little about me before you read on. I am a physician specializing in internal medicine and have been employed for two years at the Department of Infectious Diseases at Rigshospitalet, a national university hospital in Denmark. I have passed a three-month course in tropical medicine and became a professor in clinical research design and analysis in 2010. I cofounded the Cochrane Collaboration in 1993, which is an organization that has published over 10,000 systematic reviews or protocols for upcoming reviews about the benefits and harms of interventions in healthcare. My only aim in relation to vaccines, as in any other area of healthcare, is to get as close to the truth as I can. Being a scientist, I do not "take sides." I study the evidence and base my conclusions on what I find, regardless of the consequences for myself. My criticism of the prestigious Cochrane review of the HPV vaccines was an important reason why I was expelled from Cochrane in 2018 after a show trial, which I have described in my book *Death of a Whistleblower and Cochrane's Moral Collapse*.[16]

Pervasive Misinformation on the Internet

There is substantial misinformation about vaccines on the Internet. A 2019 search for *vaccine* on Amazon showed that 15 of the 18 books and movies listed on the search page had vaccine-denying content.[17] There were books and movies that made their stance clear already in their titles, e.g., the movies *We Don't Vaccinate!* and *Shoot 'Em Up: The Truth About Vaccines*.

The algorithms that power social media platforms as well as Amazon's recommendations are not designed to distinguish quality information from misinformation. Therefore, harmful messages have been able to thrive and spread.

As another example, Facebook's autofill suggestions for *vaccine* steers users toward misinformation.[18] Even if using a neutral search term, such as *vaccination*, the results are dominated by vaccine-denying propaganda: the top 12 groups were all against vaccines, led by two misinformation groups, *Stop Mandatory Vaccination* and *Vaccination Re-education Discussion Forum*, with more than 140,000 members each. Facebook accepts advertising, boosting the misinformation further. The ads from *Stop Mandatory Vaccination* have included blatantly false statements such as "vaccines kill babies."

On YouTube, owned by Google, users seeking information about vaccines are similarly nudged toward misinformation, much of it designed to frighten parents. Even when users find scientifically sound content, such as a video uploaded by the Mayo Clinic (the top search result for *MMR vaccine*), YouTube's "up next" algorithm recommends users to watch a vaccine-denying video.[19] Critics have also pointed to YouTube's practice of recommending videos based on watch history, which leads users to misinformation.

Both Facebook and YouTube have begun treating misinformation that can lead to harm as a special category meriting additional scrutiny and mitigation. In the meantime, the harms of vaccine misinformation continue. A recent UK study found that half of all parents with small children were exposed to misinformation about vaccines on social media.[20] Half of all parents!

The pervasive misinformation has dire consequences. Many people—including our most defenseless citizens, our children—have died unnecessarily because of it.

The scientists have lost the PR war to quacks and fraudsters. I have browsed many homepages and have noticed that many people—including doctors—have made fortunes by their deadly misinformation. Some doctors are even against using antibiotics, and some tell people that, instead of getting vaccinated, they should use homeopathy, which is bogus, as there isn't a single active molecule in it, or to eat some fancy supplements or herbs they happen to sell themselves that don't work, either.[21] Many quacks describe themselves as being holistic. After having challenged some of them to explain what they mean by this, I have realized that it is a euphemism for saying: "I don't know what I am doing, but it surely gives me a huge income to fool people."

According to the editors of the *New York Times*, the "anti-vaxxers" have hundreds of websites promoting their messages, a roster of tech- and media-savvy influencers, and an aggressive political arm that includes at least a dozen political action committees.[22] The "defense against this onslaught has been meagre," and the few academics that try to counterargue the pseudo-science with fact get bombarded with vitriol, including outright threats.[23]

In 2015, a team of US researchers analyzed 480 "anti-vaccine" websites.[24] They were seriously misleading: 66% claimed that vaccines are dangerous, 62% that they cause autism, and 41% that they cause brain injury. Websites often used anecdotes to support these claims.

Commonly copromoted behaviors include the use of alternative medicine (19%), homeopathy (10%), eating a healthy (19%) or organic (5%) diet, and cleansing one's body of toxins (7%). This is bogus.[25] Nothing in the world can add anything to the excellent detoxifying organs we have, the liver and the kidneys. There is more. Closed groups on Facebook are fed false information, often by people with a clear financial interest in discrediting vaccines.[26] By barring access to others, they are able to serve undiluted misinformation without being challenged. The groups are large and sophisticated, e.g., as just noted, *Stop Mandatory Vaccination* has more than 140,000 approved members.

Vitamin C & Orthomolecular Medicine for Optimal Health tells its users that it is "not an anti-vax group." Yet anyone allowed into this closed group of about 49,000 approved members will find ample material questioning the safety of vaccines. There are also recommendations for alternative remedies that are falsely claimed to protect against disease. The group's leader, Katie Gironda, is CEO of an online business in Colorado selling high-dose vitamin C. Members of her closed group are encouraged to "shop now"—in one click they are linked directly to her firm, *Revitalize Wellness*. The site sells vitamin C powder in bulk, and customers are encouraged to give two-year-old children up to three grams a day. This is very dangerous. The recommended daily intake is only 15 mg, and vitamin C has many harms. Google *vitamin C side effects* and you will see. According to the Mayo Clinic, "High doses of vitamin C have been associated with multiple adverse effects. These include blood clotting, death (heart-related), kidney stones, pro-oxidant effects, problems with the digestive system, and red blood cell destruction."[27] There are many fraudsters on the Vitamin C market who say that the vitamin can cure virtually everything, including cancer, heart disease, tuberculosis, and the deadly viral disease Ebola.[28]

Revitalize Wellness carries a disclaimer saying its products are "not intended to treat, diagnose, cure or prevent disease."[29] But in conversation with members of her closed Facebook group, Gironda gives the opposite advice: "Vitamin C has an amazing record of fighting the same diseases vaccines were made for." This statement is totally false. In another entry she says that she avoids all vaccines.

Gironda is also listed as an administrator of a separate Facebook group called *Vitamin C Against Vaccine Damage*, where she claims that "Vitamin C is the safest and most effective way to protect from damage for those that are mandated to be vaccinated." After *The Guardian* contacted Gironda, the status of the group *Vitamin C Against Vaccine Damage* was changed from closed to secret. That put it into an even more heavily shrouded category that hides the group entirely from the view of nonmembers by taking it out of Facebook searches.

It deserves to be repeated that all such misinformation has the potential to kill children and has very likely done so.

In addition to hosting many closed anti-vaccination groups, Facebook has taken in thousands of advertising dollars from those who specifically target parents, often with frightening and false messages meant to undermine trust in vaccines.

The arguments used by people driving the anti-vaccination movement have not changed in about a century. They are effective because they are intuitively appealing, but they are easily refutable. Instead of ignoring them, an effective pro-vaccine campaign should confront them directly, over and over, for as long as it takes.[30]

The most successful vaccines are victims of their own success. They have beaten so many infectious foes into oblivion that hardly any practicing doctors, let alone new parents, remember how terrible those diseases once were.[31] In most countries, we have not only eliminated smallpox, diphtheria, polio, and measles (it was declared eradicated in the United States in 2000 but has since come back), but we have also eliminated the memory of these diseases.

Deaths and Other Serious Harms with and without Vaccines

We live in a world that is so overdiagnosed and overtreated that, in high-income countries, our medications are the third-leading cause of death after heart disease and cancer. This has been demonstrated in several independent studies in Europe and North America.[32] Based on the best research I could find, I have estimated that psychiatric drugs alone are also the third leading cause of death.[33] It might not be that bad, but psychiatric drugs do take many lives, and yet over 10% of the population in many countries take at least one psychiatric drug every day.

Drugs are a double-edged sword, and most of them are unspecific and have a range of effects in addition to the intended one, many of which are harmful. We should therefore use drugs as little as possible to protect ourselves against death and other harms.

Vaccines are totally different. They are highly specific, directed against one microorganism, need only to be used once or a few times, usually provide many years of protection or even life-long immunity, serious harms are very rare, and it is usually vastly cheaper to get vaccinated than to take drugs. These properties make vaccines the most valuable interventions and the best buy for the money we can offer in healthcare. They are also vastly safer, on average, than other drugs.

Among all the good vaccines, the measles vaccine is one of those that has saved the most lives. It therefore does not make sense that vaccine deniers consider the measles vaccine their main target.

During the US measles outbreak in 2014–2015, unsubstantiated claims of deaths caused by the MMR vaccine began circulating on the Internet. They were based on spontaneous reports submitted to the US Vaccine Adverse Event Reporting System (VAERS).[34] Some vaccine-denying groups even postulated that more deaths were caused by the MMR vaccine than by measles, which is an absurd comparison, as the reason that so few people die from measles is that almost the whole population is vaccinated. The title of an article in *Newsweek* is telling: "A look at anti-vaxxers' monstrously bad measles math."[35]

In contrast to these unwarranted scare campaigns, an in-depth review of the VAERS data by physicians from the FDA and the CDC showed that many of the deaths involved children with serious preexisting medical conditions or were likely unrelated to vaccination (e.g., accidents). No concerning patterns emerged that would suggest that the MMR vaccine caused deaths.[36]

It is important to realize that voluntary reporting systems accept any submitted report of an adverse event without judging whether it was caused by a vaccine. The function of passive surveillance systems is to detect signals and generate hypotheses about possible adverse effects of vaccines and other drugs. It requires expertise in research methods and other knowledge to analyze the reports and arrive at tentative conclusions about cause-effect relationships. As an example, media attention related to the discredited hypothesis that measles vaccines can cause autism may lead to an increase in reports on autism, thereby creating a false impression that the incidence is related to increasing use of vaccination.

In 2015, people employed by the CDC published a comprehensive review of deaths following vaccination.[37]

In 1955, an error in the Salk polio vaccine manufacturing process led to production of a vaccine that, although aimed at being inactivated, contained live poliovirus.[38] This resulted in one of the worst vaccine disasters in history, with 40,000 cases of polio resulting in 51 cases of paralysis and five deaths among vaccinated people. In addition, there were 113 cases of paralysis and five deaths among contacts of vaccinated people. As a result, the US government implemented much more vigilant monitoring and regulation of the vaccine industry.

It should be noted that back then, regulation of drugs was very poor.[39] In the first half of the twentieth century, there weren't any demands that drugs should have been demonstrated to have a therapeutic or prophylactic effect. What was most important was that they were not unduly harmful, and not even that was adequately investigated. As a result, several drug catastrophes occurred, and many dangerous drugs were withdrawn from the market after having harmed or killed many people. The thalidomide disaster, where a sleeping pill caused horrible birth defects leading to loss of limbs, led to important changes in drug regulation, and this drug was withdrawn in 1962.[40]

In rare cases, vaccines cause autoimmune diseases. These occur because people with certain tissue types have antigens (receptors) that resemble the antigens in the vaccines. Therefore, the intentional stimulation of the immune system leads to production of antibodies both against the virus or bacterium and against people's own tissues.

This mechanism is not limited to vaccines. Infections, and other foreign agents, can also cause autoimmune diseases. Thus, a suspected harm of a vaccine may merely be the result of a concomitant infection, which might have passed unnoticed. The suspicion of vaccine-induced harm is considerably heightened if rechallenge, e.g., second or third immunizations with the same vaccine, produces the same or worse symptoms.

A single study, no matter how carefully designed, cannot usually be taken as definitive evidence that a vaccine causes a certain harm. Manipulations with the data are common in medical research, and fraud also occurs, which is why we need more than one study.

The results of multiple large reviews and studies have been reassuring. In 2011, the US Institute of Medicine produced an 866-page report based on over 12,000 articles about adverse events reported after vaccines.[41] There was convincing evidence of 14 adverse events being caused by vaccines, which occurred very rarely. The vaccine strain virus was isolated in disseminated Oka varicella zoster virus infection and in encephalitis caused by the MMR vaccine caused by the measles component. The MMR vaccine can cause febrile seizures, and anaphylaxis (allergic shock) was seen after six vaccines (MMR, varicella, influenza, hepatitis B, meningococcal, and tetanus). Injection of any vaccine can lead to syncope (fainting) and deltoid bursitis. It is also well established that the oral polio vaccine on rare occasions causes paralytic polio.

Less firm conclusions about a causal relationship were drawn for HPV vaccine and anaphylaxis, MMR vaccine and transient arthralgia, and certain trivalent influenza vaccines used in Canada and a mild, temporary oculorespiratory syndrome. For many other adverse events, it was unclear whether there was a causal relationship.

* * *

In 1994, the US Institute of Medicine published a review of deaths reported to VAERS after childhood vaccinations.[42] The vast majority of reported deaths were coincidental and not causally related to the vaccines. There was only one death due to a vaccine strain viral infection: a 3-month-old infant died from myocarditis after an oral polio vaccine; as the virus was isolated from the child's heart, this was the likely cause.

In another review of deaths reported to VAERS in the 1990s, nearly half of the deaths were due to sudden infant death syndrome. The death rate fell after people were advised to let their babies sleep on their backs instead of on their tummies. Deaths from other causes also declined even though the number of vaccines administered increased.

A study published in 2013 reviewed health information from over 13 million vaccinated persons and compared causes of death in the vaccinated study population to the general US population. The death rate 1–2 months following vaccination was lower than that in the population, and the causes of death were similar.[43] This study provides convincing evidence that vaccinations are not associated with an increased risk of death.

However, there are rare instances where causal relationships between vaccination and death have been established or a plausible theoretical risk exists.[44]

Anaphylaxis following Vaccination
Anaphylaxis is a serious allergic reaction that can be caused by many things, including drugs and bee stings. The risk of anaphylaxis is very low, less than two cases per million doses of vaccines administered to children and adolescents, but people who have just been vaccinated should be observed for 15 minutes, and healthcare providers should be prepared to treat anaphylaxis with adrenaline, which can be life-saving. A 10-year review of claims to the US National Vaccine Injury Compensation Program noted only five deaths from anaphylaxis after vaccinations.

Severely Immunocompromised Persons Receiving Live Vaccines
Live vaccine viruses are attenuated so they do not cause infection in people with intact immune systems, but they are contraindicated for people who are severely immunocompromised. Two severely immunocompromised children died after a varicella vaccine, and six persons died after a measles vaccine.

Intussusception after Rotavirus Vaccine
Intussusception is a rare medical condition in which the bowel folds in, or telescopes, on itself. It is a type of ileus (arrest of bowel movements). The first licensed rotavirus vaccine, which is used to prevent diarrhea, was withdrawn from use in 1999 after a greater than expected number of reports of intussusception were detected in postmarketing surveillance. Only one death was reported. It has been estimated that the currently used vaccines prevent 70 deaths for every death they cause. A published review of VAERS reports for 2006–2012 found two deaths from intussusception, but a definitive causal association with vaccination was not established.

Guillain–Barré Syndrome after Inactivated Influenza Vaccines
In 1976, concerns in the United States about a possible influenza pandemic involving a virus similar to the deadly 1918 pandemic strain resulted in a large-scale vaccination program. The US government stopped the program when no swine flu cases were detected outside the military base where the disease originated and when an unexpectedly high number of cases of the Guillain-Barré syndrome were reported. This is an autoimmune disease characterized by damage to the peripheral nervous system, which leads to changes in sensation and pain, and to muscle weakness, which may progress to paralysis, also of the respiratory muscles, and death. The vaccine

was estimated to have caused approximately one Guillain-Barré syndrome case per 100,000 persons vaccinated, resulting in 53 deaths.

Studies assessing the risk of Guillain-Barré syndrome after seasonal inactivated influenza vaccine since 1976 have shown either no risk or a very small risk of 1–2 cases per million doses. One study found that the risk over the entire influenza season was lower in people who received the 2009 vaccines compared to unvaccinated people. Another study, based on electronic health record data from 2000 through 2009, reported two deaths, but a causal relation with vaccination was not established.

Thus, it is not clear whether current influenza vaccines cause deaths related to the Guillain-Barré syndrome.

Fainting after Vaccination Leading to Head Trauma and Death
Needle sticks for any reason can lead to fainting. In a study on quadrivalent human papillomavirus vaccine (HPV) among young women, 15% reported fainting or near-fainting after the first dose. A VAERS case report described a death after head trauma following a fall that occurred some minutes after vaccination with a hepatitis B vaccine.

Paralytic Poliomyelitis from Oral Poliovirus Vaccine
In the United States, from 1980 to 1989, there were two deaths. The live attenuated oral polio vaccine is no longer used in the United States, where it has been replaced with inactivated poliovirus vaccine, whereas it is used in many other countries because it is cheaper than the inactivated one.

Conflicts of Interest in Organizations Recommending Vaccines

Some prominent vaccine advocacy organizations are pushing for greater compulsion.[45] All US states require vaccination as a condition for school entry, and in 2015, California followed Mississippi and West Virginia and passed a law removing the personal belief exemption that had previously allowed families to defer or decline mandated childhood vaccinations. Every Child By Two and the American Academy of Pediatrics supported the bill. Immunization Action Coalition, another major vaccine advocacy organization, runs one of the web's most visited sites for free vaccine information for healthcare providers. It advocates for increasing rates of influenza vaccination among healthcare workers through mandates, maintaining an "influenza vaccination honor roll" of more than 600 organizations as "stellar examples of influenza vaccination mandates in healthcare settings."

These three organizations are all nonprofit and have large online presences that promote themselves as sources of reliable information on vaccines. However, they receive funding from vaccine manufacturers and from the CDC. Furthermore, in their advocacy for compulsory vaccination, they all push beyond official governmental policy and, in the case of influenza vaccines, beyond the evidence.[46] When challenged by the *BMJ*, the Immunization Action Coalition noted: "While there is debate and research directed at assessing the nature and degree of benefit that vaccinating healthcare workers confers to patients, we are not aware of any definitive and universally accepted study showing a complete lack of benefit." This sheer nonsense reverses the burden of proof. Furthermore, scientifically, it is impossible to show that something *does not* exist. Philosopher Bertrand Russell once wrote that we cannot be certain that there isn't a porcelain tea set circulating in orbit. No, we cannot be certain, but is it likely?

There is a tangled web between the three organizations and the CDC, which makes it very difficult to find out where the money comes from, and how much, also because the amounts are rarely declared.[47] It almost looks like whitewashing, as we know it from numerous bank scandals. The CDC website does not provide any clear account of the money it spends on vaccine advocacy, but it does partner with various organizations and has donated, for example, over $2 million to the Immunization Action Coalition since 2009 to help increase vaccination rates by creating "external sources of scientific, accurate, and credible immunization information that healthcare providers can use to communicate with parents and the public." Considering the massive amount of misinformation the CDC provides about influenza vaccines (see Chapter 4), this announcement looks like a joke.

None of the three organizations has ever questioned a CDC recommendation. According to Barbara Mintzes, who does research on conflicts of interest:

> these groups are so strongly pro-vaccination that the public is getting a
> one-sided message that all vaccines are created equal and vaccination is an
> important public health strategy, regardless of the circumstances. This is
> as unhelpful as an 'anti-vaxxer' approach that assumes all vaccinations are
> harmful. Reality is a little different: Some vaccines are enormously important
> to public health; others are marginal at best and likely best avoided.[48]

There are also conflicts of interest in drug agencies, at WHO and other national and international institutions, and I shall discuss some of these in the following chapters.

Only about 10% of WHO's budget is covered by member state fees; the rest is supplied by public and private partners.[49] The 90% donated by the partners influences WHO policies, as only about 5% of the voluntary contributions are for core activities; the rest is earmarked for specific projects.

The founder of Microsoft, Bill Gates, contributes almost half a billion dollars annually to the WHO, or over one-fifth of the donations, via the Bill and Melinda Gates Foundation and the GAVI Alliance (which he launched in 2000 under the name Global Alliance for Vaccines and Immunization). One of the aims is to collect donations from rich countries to help third-world governments procure vaccines.[50]

These praiseworthy initiatives have side effects. The focus on vaccination can detract attention from other important health issues such as pollution, contaminated water, lack of sewerage, and poverty. In 2008, the director of the WHO program against malaria turned to WHO's director general to denounce the "enormous, largely undesirable consequences" that the Gates funding had on his research area.[51] The scientists were imprisoned in a cartel of funding that made independent review of the studies increasingly difficult. And he warned that the foundation's determination to have its favored research used to guide its recommendations could have untoward consequences for the policy-making process.

Bill Gates is known for being very industry friendly and supportive of patents. Gates's approach has been criticized by Doctors without Borders because it focuses on introducing new expensive vaccines—rather than shifting to a stronger emphasis on improving basic health services and immunizations with cheap vaccines.[52]

2

Measles

For the last 20 years, measles has been the primary target in the battles between vaccine advocates and vaccine deniers. I shall demonstrate what is right and what is wrong.

It is important to understand that the difference between survival and death depends on the infectious dose. Peter Aaby's studies in Africa and elsewhere have disproved the prevailing dogma that malnourishment plays a significant role for measles mortality.[1] By using Danish patient files from 1915 to 1925, he confirmed his initial findings from the tropics that the more children there are in a family, the higher the death rate during measles epidemics.[2] He concluded that this is because overcrowding results in more intensive exposure within families, transferring greater doses of the virus. The children died before they had mounted an effective immune response. This explains why measles outbreaks can be particularly deadly in countries experiencing a natural disaster or conflict, with overcrowding in refugee camps that not only greatly increases the risk of infection,[3] but also the risk of dying from it.

Aaby's findings were met with great disbelief by the establishment, but they are highly convincing. They are over 30 years old and have now been generally accepted, but dogmas have a life of their own, and a whole generation of doctors impregnated with false information needs to die out before the dogmas—perhaps—disappear for good. One can still find the erroneous idea about malnourishment in articles and textbooks, e.g., in a so-called fact sheet from WHO from 2018: "Severe measles is more likely among poorly nourished young children."[4]

After having studied the science, I have come to the conclusion that the measles vaccine is one of the best interventions we have in healthcare. It is very strange that it is necessary to remind people about this. But the sad fact is that some people—including physicians and other well-educated people who should know better—refuse to vaccinate their children against measles.

I have tried to understand the vaccine deniers' reasoning and will discuss their most important arguments below. Even in hard-core groups, there may be people who can be influenced by rational arguments, good science, and ethical deliberations, particularly if you can demonstrate that what they have believed in is based on false information.

A Canceled Meeting in California

It was with this hope in mind that I accepted to speak at a meeting in California on March, 17, 2019, arranged by Physicians for Informed Consent. My talk was: "How mandatory vaccination violates medical ethics."

However, as soon as it became known that I was coming, I was subjected to a public smear campaign. I was flabbergasted. I have often been harassed when I tried to speak truth to power, but this was close to the moral bottom of what I have endured.

Social media are a paradise for people behaving like kings or high priests feeling entitled to tell everybody what they should and shouldn't do. The worst of them fire so many comments on Twitter and Facebook that they cannot have written all of it themselves, at the same time as they have a full-time job to tend to. They have an army of trolls or they are on industry payroll and publish in their own name what the drug companies have written up for them.

One of the uncrowned kings, physician David Gorski, wrote: "Holy crap @PGtzsche1, formerly of @CochraneNordic, has gone full on antivax. Here he is scheduled to speak at a workshop for the antivax doctors group with the Orwellian name Physicians for Informed Consent."[5]

On social media, many people show their worst sides and condemn others without even knowing what the issue is about. As I had never held such a talk before, Gorski could have no idea what I had decided to talk about, or what my motives and background were. He said that I would appear with "hard core antivaxers." This primitive trick is called guilt by association: "The bottom line is that @PGtzsche1 had become an antivaccine crank and deserves to be dismissed as such."[6]

As I had not been informed about who the other speakers were, I reminded the organizer about this omission:

"I asked to see the full program two weeks ago but have not seen it and I cannot find it on your home page. This is urgent as I am now attacked because I come to speak at your meeting. Some people have found out who some of the other speakers are and I am accused of being an 'anti-vaxxer,' which has nothing to do with my scientific and ethical position."

I received the program the same day and wrote back:

"I am terribly sorry, but I will have to cancel my participation immediately. You had not informed me about who the other speakers are, so I did not know what I bought into, but I have now investigated a little. One of the speakers does not vaccinate anyone although she is a doctor, another exonerates Wakefield. This is so totally anti-science and shocking to me that I cannot afford to present in such company. Sorry. I will pay back the advance you sent me and will bear the costs that I have had and cannot get refunded. I have used a lot of time on preparing for my talk but that is my problem, not yours. Please delete me from the program immediately. Many thanks."

The doctor who does not vaccinate is Toni Bark. She uses homeopathy. In an interview I found on the Internet, she said:

> What I notice is that children who come to me from other practices where they've been fully vaccinated often are—well they are the kids in my practice with asthma, panic disorder, OCD, pandas, autism, Asperger's. My kids who've never been vaccinated in my practice, I don't see those issues. I don't have one child who was not vaccinated who also has asthma, food allergies, or Asperger's or autism, or Crohn's or ulcerative colitis—none of these chronic, either chronic inflammatory or chronic autoimmune diseases.[7]

Bark had written to me that I should not let people like Gorski influence my decisions. I agree, but I had other concerns. In my reply, I mentioned the interview: "What you say here worries me greatly. You indicate that vaccines can cause autism, which they don't, there is no reliable evidence for this. . . . Wakefield's research is clearly fraudulent. . . . Your last sentence is like saying: I have never seen anyone die in the traffic so there cannot be any traffic accidents. This interview really scares me because your statements are seductive and lack substance. Clinical practice is hugely misleading, which is why we do RCTs [randomized clinical trials]."

Another speaker was lawyer Mary Holland, who has written that "Dr. Wakefield has joined in a long, honorable tradition of dissidents in science and human rights. The world has benefitted profoundly from other courageous dissidents in science—Galileo, who argued that the sun is the center of the universe; Semmelweis, who reasoned that doctors must wash their hands to prevent transmission of infection . . ."[8]

People like Holland do harm by spreading false messages about the science. Andrew Wakefield and his coworkers claimed that the MMR vaccine can cause autism, but a series of articles in the *British Medical Journal (BMJ)* in 2011 revealed that their research is fraudulent.[9]

The truth is that rigorous research has failed to establish any link between vaccination and autism,[10] but this doesn't mean anything for vaccine deniers, as they cannot be reached for a rational debate. An example of their dogmatism is the website "Autism Investigated." On April 13, 2019, under the headline "Robert F. Kennedy Jr. wants to preserve uncle JFK's vaccine program," they wrote that Kennedy appeared in a video in 2015 where he stated that he wants "policies that encourage full vaccination for all Americans." They opined that "Vaccine programs should not exist. They are deadly" and that Kennedy "surrounds himself with idiots, opportunists, and vaccine crime apologists." Interestingly, Gorski called Kennedy an antivaxxer. How can the same person be both for and against vaccines? This is not a problem for the kings on social media who hide their lack of arguments behind colorful and derogatory nouns and adjectives.

If we turn our backs on vaccine deniers by telling them they are foolish and dangerous, it might recruit even more deniers from the undecided crowd in the middle who might see conspiracies where there are none. I therefore still considered going to the meeting in California, also because the organizer had assured me that most of the attendants were pediatricians "who give vaccines every day, they just don't want parents to be COERCED into consenting for a vaccine under threat that their child won't be able to attend school." Furthermore, she encouraged me to criticize her published statements about the measles vaccine, which I shall do below.

A week before the meeting, I chaired an international scientific meeting I had arranged in Copenhagen, which was the inaugural symposium for the Institute for Scientific Freedom, of which I am the director. People had signed up from around the world, and my supporters were very worried that my participation in the California meeting would be used against us— guilt by association—and detract attention from what the new institute was about. One of the lectures was about vaccines, held by Peter Aaby,[11] and some highly vocal attendees at the symposium wanted so badly for the discussions after the talks to focus on vaccines that I had to stop them. They seemed to be vaccine deniers wanting to propagate their false beliefs, as if they were missionaries from a religious sect.

Wakefield's Horrendous Fraud

The vaccine deniers propagate misinformation and utter nonsense on their websites and social media, which are "liked" or copied by others acting like robots, without letting any rational thought come in the way. They gloss over Andrew Wakefield's horrendous fraud by pretending it never happened and say he was right about measles causing autism.

Incidentally, in 2016, I discovered that my portrait had appeared on the front page of the website of the US Alliance for Human Research Protection under the heading *Honors Exemplary Professionals*. Portraits of people of good repute came and went in slow succession, and I couldn't believe it when, at the end of gallery, which was in alphabetic order, I saw a photo of Wakefield. The Alliance calls itself a "national network of lay people and professionals dedicated to advancing responsible and ethical medical research practices." Wakefield is notorious for having done the opposite. I therefore asked to have my name and photo removed.

In an email to me, the founder and president of the alliance, Vera Sharav, defended Wakefield vigorously with arguments that I found were highly unlikely to be true. I therefore contacted the award-winning investigative journalist Brian Deer, who exposed Wakefield's fraud in the *Sunday Times* and the *BMJ*.[12] He sent me and Sharav an account of the issues and explained that she had copied and pasted from vaccine deniers' websites without investigating the issues herself. Much of what she wrote was plain wrong.

Sharav preferred to let me go and keep Wakefield on the honors list, where he still is. Without implying guilt by association, I don't understand why the people in Wakefield's company didn't ask to be removed. I wrote to several of them and drew their attention to Wakefield's fraud. At least two of the honorable people cannot request to be removed because they are dead; one of them, Florence Nightingale, in 1910. As I had never given my permission to be on Sharav's list, I felt abused. My credibility had been used to shine a good light on Wakefield.

Wakefield published his research fraud in the *Lancet* in 1998,[13] and Deer's revelations of it are second to none. The fraud and Wakefield's subsequent public relations campaigns have been immensely harmful. Since many people deny the facts, or don't know about them, and depict Wakefield as a hero, it is crucial in a book about vaccines to provide detail about the events.[14]

Wakefield's research was rigged right from the start. He claimed he had discovered a new syndrome, which he dubbed "autistic enterocolitis" in a paper later retracted by the *American Journal of Gastroenterology*. Wakefield claimed that the live measles vaccine caused both autism and inflammatory bowel disease, which was a result he never found but badly needed to bring his secret grand business plans to fruition.

Contrary to the rules, Wakefield did not reveal his financial conflicts of interest. While he held himself out to be a dispassionate scientist, two years before the *Lancet* paper was published—and before any of the 12 children in his study were even referred to the hospital—he had been hired to attack the MMR vaccine by a lawyer, Richard Barr, who hoped to raise a class action lawsuit against the manufacturers.

Unlike expert witnesses in court cases, Wakefield had negotiated an unprecedented contract with Barr to conduct clinical and basic research. The goal was to find evidence of what the two men claimed to be a new syndrome intended to be the centerpiece of (later failed) litigation on behalf of an eventual 1,600 British families, recruited through media stories. When Deer exposed this in 2004, it led to public uproar in Britain and the longest-ever professional misconduct hearing by the UK's General Medical Council (GMC). Barr paid Wakefield with money from the UK legal aid fund run by the government to give poor people access to justice. Wakefield charged an extraordinary amount of about $750,000, plus expenses, for generic work alone. In addition, he was awarded an initial £55,000 to conduct the research later submitted to *Lancet*.

The chief executive at the hospital where Wakefield worked wrote to him that a grant would be established for the purpose, given his written confirmation that there was no conflict of interest involved. However, when the *Lancet* paper was published, and the vaccine scare was launched at a televised press conference, nobody was aware that Wakefield was receiving substantial personal payments from Barr. Because of the expected panic, extra phone lines and answering machines had been installed, and a 23-minute video news release showcasing Wakefield's claims was distributed to broadcasters. In the video, Wakefield said that the MMR vaccine should be suspended in favor of the single vaccines.

Wakefield had filed a single vaccine patent eight months before the press conference, arguing for a "safer" single measles shot. His incentive for launching a vaccine scare and to keep it going for as long as possible was huge. A 35-page "private and confidential" prospectus noted that the initial market for a diagnostic test based on a patent Wakefield had filed in 1995 would be litigation-driven testing of patients with "autistic enterocolitis" from both the United Kingdom and the United States. The patent claimed that "Crohn's disease or ulcerative colitis may be diagnosed by detecting measles virus in bowel tissue, bowel products or body fluids." It was estimated that by year three, income from this testing could be about £3.3 million, and rising to £28 million.

Wakefield's start-up funding was part of a staggering £26 million of taxpayers' money (more than $56 million at 2014 prices) eventually shared among a small group of doctors and lawyers, working under Barr's and Wakefield's direction, trying to prove that MMR caused the previously unheard-of "syndrome." It is remarkable that Wakefield had asserted the existence of such a syndrome *before* he performed the research that purportedly discovered it. Six months before the *Lancet* report, the lawyer reminded the doctor in a confidential letter: "I have mentioned to you before that the prime objective is to produce unassailable evidence in court so as to convince a court that these vaccines are dangerous."[15]

The Barr-Wakefield deal was the foundation of the vaccine crisis throughout the world. Even as the *Lancet* paper was being prepared, behind the scenes Wakefield was negotiating extraordinary plans to exploit the public alarm with secret schemes that would line his pockets. Although Wakefield denied any such plans, confidential documents[16] set out his proposed shot, and a network of companies intended to raise venture capital for purported inventions, including a replacement for attenuated viral vaccines, commercial testing kits, and what was claimed to be a possible cure for autism.[17]

Deer discovered that nearly all the 12 children had been preselected through MMR campaign groups and that, at the time of their admission, most of their parents were clients and contacts of the lawyer, Barr. It is the most bizarre setup for "research" I have ever heard about. It is like stating the verdict in a criminal case before any evidence has been collected and without even knowing what this evidence would show or if a crime had ever been committed.

The *Lancet* paper's incredible purported finding—of a sudden onset of autism within days of vaccination—was a total sham built on unverified, vague, and sometimes altered memories and assertions of a group of unnamed parents who, unbeknownst to the journal and its readers, were bound to blame the vaccine when they came to the hospital because that was why they had been brought there. Wakefield, a former trainee gut surgeon, denied this.

There was also widespread falsification of patient selection criteria, clinical histories, and neuropsychiatric diagnoses. In not one case in the series of 12 children could the *Lancet* paper be reconciled with National Health Service records, and in not one case could the purported diagnosis of inflammatory bowel disease be confirmed. When the results of the pathological examinations were shown to others, they said that they were overwhelmingly normal and might be found in almost anybody's gut. The original slides were said to have been lost, which is the standard excuse when people face trouble in fraud cases: "Sorry, the termites ate my data!"

Unsurprisingly, the GMC panel ruled that key elements of the *Lancet* paper were intentionally dishonest. The authors had omitted from the paper the children's principal gastroenterological problem. Almost all had severe constipation, and standard blood tests for inflammation were normal, but this was also unreported. Some children were a cause for concern before vaccination. Some were deemed normal months afterward. Some did not have autism.[18]

Wakefield said he had nothing to do with the pathological findings, although the paper stated that he assessed the biopsy specimens with the pathologist and a trainee: "All tissues were assessed by three other clinical and experimental pathologists (APD, AA, AJW)"[19] (the *Lancet* paper can still be read, on *Lancet*'s website, for free; on every page is written RETRACTED in big, bold, red letters). Wakefield has since claimed that the statement is wrong—pretty curious, as he is first author of the paper and has the ultimate responsibility of ensuring that everything is correct, not least his own role.

No reputable research ethics committee would have endorsed the kind of fishing expedition Wakefield embarked on for Barr, and without that endorsement, no reputable medical journal would have published any resulting paper. Wakefield falsely reported that a grueling five-day battery of invasive and distressing procedures performed on the kids—including anesthesia, ileocolonoscopies, lumbar punctures, MRI brain scans, EEGs, radioactive drinks, and x-rays—proposed for the lawsuit was approved by the Royal Free's ethics committee.

Deer revealed that the ethics committee was not told the truth about the project and had given no such approval. Responding to Deer in 2004, Wakefield and his key associates, pediatricians John Walker-Smith and

Simon Murch, denied this explosive discovery and issued a formal statement. But, after being confronted with the proof at the GMC hearing, they changed their story and—despite clear rules—now argued they had needed no approval.[20]

The story was much the same for Wakefield's basic science. He had planned his business ventures against a theory of his own that the culprit for both inflammatory bowel disease and autism was persistent infection with measles virus, which, in an attenuated form, is found live as a normal part of MMR. But Deer revealed that sophisticated, unreported, molecular tests carried out in Wakefield's own laboratory had found no trace of measles in the children's guts or blood. There were also critical flaws in one apparently positive study, which involved materials supplied by Wakefield. This fraud misled thousands of families affected by autism, both in the United Kingdom and United States, ensnared for years in hopeless litigation based almost entirely on his measles theory.

Two years before Deer's revelations, the American Academy of Pediatrics summarized the consensus: "Numerous studies have refuted Andrew Wakefield's theory that MMR vaccine is linked to bowel disorders and autism. . . . Every aspect of Dr. Wakefield's theory has been disproven."[21] In the United States, the Barr-Wakefield deal was joined by allegations marshaled by American attorneys that a mercury-based vaccine preservative, thimerosal, was also at fault (see below).

In response to Deer, Wakefield supporters have denied that he took money for research and, amid a barrage of sometimes paid-for smears and crank abuse of Deer, lauded the doctor as a "hero." Wakefield's deceits not only triggered the resurgence of sometimes fatal or brain-damaging measles outbreaks; they also plunged countless parents into the hell of believing it was their own fault for agreeing to vaccination that a son or daughter developed autism.

Wakefield denied any conflicts of interest and claimed he never said that MMR caused autism. But documents—including patents—evidenced this, and he published a string of falsified reports to undermine the vaccine. Even when he knew that his allegations had been proven baseless, he was found promoting them from a controversial business in Austin, Texas, where—after being fired from the Royal Free in October 2001—he held a $280,000-a-year post, spun from his campaign.

Throughout the investigation, Wakefield refused to cooperate, filed baseless complaints, and issued statements denying every aspect. He also initiated, sought to stall, and then abandoned with some £1.3 million

($2 million) costs a two-year "gagging" libel lawsuit, financed by the Medical Protection Society, which defends doctors against their patients. In reply, Deer and Channel 4 pressed for a speedy trial, publicly accusing Wakefield of being "unremittingly evasive and dishonest."[22] His conduct in the litigation was also damned by a High Court judge, who said that Wakefield wished to extract whatever advantage he could from the existence of the proceedings, while not wishing to progress them, and that he was using the lawsuit as a weapon in his attempts to close down discussion and debate over an important public issue.

Faced with overwhelming proof of misconduct, Wakefield concocted a preposterous conspiracy theory to account for his exposure and to explain why he could not reveal what he called "vaccine secrets." He also denied rigging his results. "The notion that any researcher can cook such data in any fashion that can be slipped past the medical community for his personal benefit is patent nonsense," he argued in a March 2009 statement. "Mr. Deer's implications of fraud against me are claims that a trained physician and researcher of good standing had suddenly decided he was going to fake data for his own enrichment."[23]

On January 28, 2010—after 197 days of evidence, submissions, and deliberations—a panel of three doctors and two lay members hearing the GMC case handed down verdicts that wholly vindicated Deer. Branding Wakefield "dishonest," "unethical," and "callous," they found him guilty (against a criminal standard of proof) of some three dozen charges, including four counts of dishonesty and 12 involving the abuse of developmentally challenged children.[24] His research was found to be dishonest and performed without ethical approval. Five days later, Lancet retracted the paper as "utterly false," prompting international media interest and further retractions.

Three weeks later, on February 17, 2010, Wakefield was ousted by the directors of his Texas business, and he was later erased from the UK doctors' register, ending his career in medicine.

Lancet editor-in-chief Richard Horton protected Wakefield. In 2004, after four months of investigations, Deer briefed Lancet's senior staff for five hours. Later the same day, he discussed the affair with Horton and five other editors. Deer had expected Horton to say that an investigation was needed to untangle the complex matters, including possible research fraud, unethical treatment of vulnerable children, and Wakefield's conflict of interest through the lawyer. But within 48 hours, and working with the paper's three senior authors, the journal produced an avalanche of denials in statements they never retracted.[25]

Wakefield arrived at the *Lancet* before Deer left the building. All three senior authors were former Royal Free staff, as was Horton—a fellow in the late 1980s. A decade before Wakefield's publication, Horton had done research in hepatology, on the same corridor as Wakefield in gastroenterology.

"I do not regret publishing the original Wakefield paper," Horton said in a 2003 book, at the height of the UK vaccine scare. "Progress in medicine depends on the free expression of new ideas. In science, it was only this commitment to free expression that shook free the tight grip of religion on the way human beings understood their world."[26]

Horton developed his position in March 2010, after the GMC panel's findings fully endorsed what Deer had told him: "We asked the institution where the work was conducted—the Royal Free hospital—to complete an investigation. . . . They did, and they cleared Wakefield of wrongdoing."[27] But documents, emails, and replies obtained under the Freedom of Information Act revealed no formal investigation. What emerged was merely a scramble to discredit Deer's claims during the 48 hours after he disclosed the information. The documents showed that Horton, the paper's senior authors, and the Royal Free medical school frantically mobilized against Deer. Were it not for the GMC case, which cost a rumored £6 million ($9 million), Wakefield's fraud would likely forever have been denied and covered up.

The denial began as soon as Deer left the Lancet on February 18, 2004. In Horton's private office, the doctors shared their thoughts and devised a strategy. Wakefield admitted only being retained for a lawsuit and denied receiving money himself, and the pediatric gastroenterologists Walker-Smith and Murch also denied impropriety. They also denied that some children were solicited, rather than spontaneously referred, and that there was no ethical approval. In short, the accused were investigating themselves, an investigation that Horton said "cleared Wakefield."[28]

However, only 17 days later, on March 6, 2004, 10 of Wakefield's 11 coauthors (they were unable to get in contact with one of them), including Walker-Smith and Murch, published what they called a "Retraction of an interpretation":

> We wish to make it clear that in this paper no causal link was established between MMR vaccine and autism as the data were insufficient. However, the possibility of such a link was raised and consequent events have had major implications for public health. In view of this, we consider now is the

appropriate time that we should together formally retract the interpretation placed upon these findings in the paper, according to precedent.[29]

It took the *Lancet* six more years, or 12 years in total, to retract the fraudulent paper. When Wakefield refused to carry out the replication research requested of him by his employers, they fired him.

In January 2011, *BMJ*'s editor-in-chief called Wakefield's research "an elaborate fraud" and accused the Royal Free medical school and *Lancet* of "institutional and editorial misconduct."[30] Although the GMC had found Wakefield guilty of some three dozen charges, the *Lancet* continued to cover up for him. The *BMJ* editors wrote about this:

> The *Lancet* paper has of course been retracted, but for far narrower misconduct than is now apparent. The retraction statement cites the GMC's findings that the patients were not consecutively referred and the study did not have ethical approval, leaving the door open for those who want to continue to believe that the science, flawed though it always was, still stands. We hope that declaring the paper a fraud will close that door for good.[31]

Wakefield's fraud had both immediate and long-term consequences. In England, parents refused the MMR vaccine for their children, and the vaccination rates dropped from 91% in 1998 to below 80% in 2003.[32]

There were measles outbreaks in London, which quickly spread to Scotland and Ireland. In 2002, 100 children in Ireland were hospitalized with measles-associated bronchopneumonia or acute encephalitis, and three children died from measles encephalitis. Another child died of measles complications in England during a 2006 outbreak.

Vaxxed: From Cover-up to Catastrophe, a Catastrophically Bad Film Directed by Wakefield

Is Wakefield still around and still being harmful? Very much so. By 2009, one in five parents in the United States believed that vaccines cause autism.[33]

In 2016, the film *Vaxxed: From Cover-up to Catastrophe* was released. This is the information about the film on its homepage, vaxxedthemovie. com:

> In 2013, biologist Dr. Brian Hooker received a call from a Senior Scientist at the U.S. Centers for Disease Control and Prevention (CDC) who led the

agency's 2004 study on the Measles-Mumps-Rubella (MMR) vaccine and its link to autism.

The scientist, Dr. William Thompson, confessed that the CDC had omitted crucial data in their final report that revealed a causal relationship between the MMR vaccine and autism. Over several months, Dr. Hooker records the phone calls made to him by Dr. Thompson who provides the confidential data destroyed by his colleagues at the CDC.

Dr. Hooker enlists the help of Dr. Andrew Wakefield, the British gastro-enterologist falsely accused of starting the anti-vax movement when he first reported in 1998 that the MMR vaccine may cause autism. In his ongoing effort to advocate for children's health, Wakefield directs this documentary examining the evidence behind an appalling cover-up committed by the government agency charged with protecting the health of American citizens.

Interviews with pharmaceutical insiders, doctors, politicians, and parents of vaccine-injured children reveal an alarming deception that has contributed to the skyrocketing increase of autism and potentially the most catastrophic epidemic of our lifetime.

The film's two main claims are that the MMR vaccine causes autism and that the CDC committed fraud to avoid revealing that their own study had shown this. If this had been true, it would have been a good film that would have won many prizes. But as both premises are wrong, it can best be described as an anti-vaccine propaganda film.

As noted earlier, it is understandable that parents to severely autistic children who were healthy before they developed autism are looking for an explanation. Autism can be totally devastating. The most well-known symptoms are extreme difficulty coping with unexpected change to routine or the environment and narrow interests in very specific topics. The restrictive behaviors tend to distance the patients from the world around them, with very limited desire to participate in social interactions. There are also repetitive behaviors, which may consist of repetitive body movements like hand flapping, rocking, spinning, moving constantly, obsessive attachment to unusual objects like rubber bands and light switches, speaking the same phrase again and again, and great distress or difficulty with changing focus. There can be abnormal body posturing or facial expressions, abnormal tone of voice, flat or monotonous speech, avoidance of eye contact, deficits in language comprehension, and delay in learning to speak. The most severely affected patients require substantial support.

I assume that the film's producer, medical journalist Del Bigtree, believed in what he was doing, but this is no excuse, as a journalist has an obligation to be objective and impartial and to check his sources. His account on the film's homepage of why he made it is telling about the drivers of the "anti-vaxx" movement.

Bigtree writes that Wakefield is "arguably the most controversial figure in modern medicine" but says he was alerted that a senior scientist from CDC, Dr. William Thompson, had confessed on the Internet that he and five colleagues had committed fraud on their 2004 MMR vaccine study when they covered up the fact that the vaccine was causally associated with autism. In Bigtree's view, the evidence was undeniable and the "CDC appeared to have lied to the world." Bigtree referred to Thompson when alleging that "during the study highly significant increases in the risk of autism were found in several distinct populations and the CDC did everything from kicking children off the study to throwing data out in order to cover it up."

Bigtree explains that without Wakefield, this story would never have been exposed.

Bigtree was surprised to find that the allegations against Wakefield were initiated "by a freelance journalist named Brian Deer who wrote a *Sunday Times* article for Rupert Murdoch that was as scientifically accurate as a gossip column." Bigtree also criticized that the General Medical Council in the United Kingdom stripped Wakefield of his medical license and he found it absurd to claim that Wakefield had used fake data to create a fraudulent paper considering that he had twelve coauthors.

Bigtree disputes that Wakefield performed unnecessary procedures on innocent children and opines that the parents had brought their children to the hospital because their children were suffering from agonizing gastrointestinal pain and bowel issues in addition to their autism.

Bigtree likens Wakefield to Galileo, who was also persecuted, and writes that "we may be responsible for a civilization-ending epidemic of autism that has skyrocketed from 1 in 10,000 to 1 in 45 children in less than forty years." He notes that the increase in autism follows a perfect exponential curve and that if something is not done, one in two children born in 2032 will "be on the autism spectrum. This is an emergency of epic proportions."

If Bigtree had read Brian Deer's many revelations in the *BMJ* and the support he got from its editors and the General Medical Council,[34] it would seem impossible to write as he did on the film's homepage unless willful ignorance was involved. It is outrageous that Bigtree likens Deer's ground-breaking investigative work to a gossip column and said that he "concocted" this unfortunate obstruction of medical advancement.

Bigtree says it's absurd to think that top scientists used fake data to create a fraudulent paper. Being a producer on a medical talk show, he should know that this has happened many times, also recently. Furthermore, it is common that top scientists lend their name to papers they know little about and that one person in a team of authors committed the fraud, often without the others' knowledge.

Bigtree talks about a civilization-ending epidemic of autism. It is of course worrying that the incidence of autism is increasing, but it is nowhere near the 200-fold increase Bigtree postulates. The diagnostic criteria for autism and autism spectrum disorders have been broadened substantially over these forty years, and it is therefore impossible to claim a 200-fold increase for something that is not the same. According to the CDC, the incidence increased only 2.5 times from 2000 to 2014, and the true increase is likely much smaller because media campaigns and increased public attention also among doctors can increase psychiatric diagnoses considerably. It would be more interesting to know if there has been any increase in the most severe cases, which will always be diagnosed.

The film makes much of a prediction done by a computer scientist who says that if the current exponential growth in the number of diagnoses continues, then 80% of boys will be autistic by 2032. Any higher bets? Why not extrapolate a few years more and arrive at 100%?

Contrary to Bigtree's prediction, the drug industry has not organized an army of bloggers to defend the vaccine. It is the vaccine deniers that have polluted the Internet.

The So-Called CDC Whistleblower Was Not a Smoking Gun

Bigtree says that Thompson found highly significant increases in the risk of autism in several distinct populations. The whole film builds on this theme, which is apparent even in its last acknowledgment: "Deepest gratitude to Dr. William Thompson. An Autism Media Channel Film 2016."

The film would collapse entirely if Thompson's claim weren't true. And it isn't true. I searched for his so-called whistleblowing on Google but did not find anything important. No facts, only opinions by vaccine deniers, which increased my suspicion that the storytelling was wrong. On psychiatrist Kelly Brogan's website, I found this:

As parents around the world have known for 7 decades [sic; 70 years], and basic science has supported, **vaccines do cause autism** [sic; in bold]. . . After Dr. Brian Hooker's requests through the Freedom of Information Act for original MMR study documentation, a CDC Immunization Safety Researcher, Dr. William Thompson has buckled under the pressure of his conscience and come forth as a whistleblower. These documents demonstrated a 3.4-fold increase in the incidence of autism in African American boys, expunged from the final study results in a violent act of scientific fraud. . . Dr. Hooker has published the unadulterated finding here.[35]

"Here" was a link to Hooker's study. Brogan did not mention that it had been retracted and was labeled as such!

It is difficult to understand all the fuss about the CDC study. It is not particularly interesting, but the way in which it was abused in the film is interesting. After having seen the film and read the paper about the study, I must say that the whole edifice for the film collapsed. The study was well done. The researchers did a case-control study in Atlanta where they matched 624 children with autism to 1,824 control children without autism.[36] The assumption for their study was that, if the MMR vaccine increases the risk of autism, which usually develops before 24 months of age, then children who are vaccinated at younger ages would have a higher risk of developing autism. They did not find this. The overall distributions of ages at first MMR vaccination were similar for case and control children (p = 0.22). The researchers analyzed their data in different ways, and I find their results very convincing.

So, what did Hooker do? He got access to the study data from Thompson and went on a fishing expedition, guided by Thompson. In research, this is considered a forbidden exploration in the data when the overall result is negative. If anything is found, it is extremely likely to be spurious.

Hooker reported in 2014 that there was a relationship between MMR timing and autism incidence among African American children "exclusively found in boys," with a risk ratio (also called the relative risk) of 1.73 (95% confidence interval 1.09 to 2.77) at 24 months and 3.36 (1.50 to 7.51) at 36 months.[37] This research is utterly hopeless.

First, there cannot be risk ratios in a case-control study, only odds ratios, which is also what the CDC had reported on.[38]

Second, black boys are a subgroup of a subgroup, which is fishing to the extreme.

Third, the confidence intervals are wide, and the lower limit is close to one. One means that there is no relation between time of vaccination and development of autism. A 95% confidence interval of 1.09 to 2.77 means that we are 95% certain that the true odds ratio is between 1.09 to 2.77.

Fourth, case-control studies are fraught with bias, which is why many respected epidemiologists have stated that, because of how easy it is to be fooled, anything less than stunning results is almost impossible to believe.[39] Some of them do not consider an increase in an odds ratio persuasive unless the lower end of the confidence interval is at least 3, which was not the case here.

Fifth, in science, one study cannot stand alone as if it were the only documentation in the universe. There are usually other studies, and in this case, some of these are much stronger. The CDC researchers refer in their discussion to six observational studies that failed to find an association between MMR vaccination and autism and consider a cohort study from Denmark particularly persuasive.[40] I agree and shall discuss it in the next section. If we want to find out if vaccination causes autism, the strongest research design is not to look at children who, with very few exceptions, all got vaccinated, as the CDC did, but to compare vaccinated with unvaccinated children and follow them up, which the Danish study did.

Although Bigtree and Wakefield were familiar with the CDC study and appear extensively in the film, neither of them mentions that much stronger studies failed to find a relation between the vaccine and autism. This is characteristic for the film, which is extremely one-sided. Its mission is to vindicate Wakefield and to tell the world how dangerous the MMR vaccine is. It is not a documentary, but sheer propaganda, which is best forgotten.

Hooker's study should also be forgotten, which quickly dawned on the editors. Only one month after publication, they retracted it, which cannot be ignored by anyone who reads it because "Retracted" is written across the abstract with big letters, and there is also a link to a note mentioning the retraction below Hooker's name:

> The Editor and Publisher regretfully retract the article as there were undeclared competing interests on the part of the author which compromised the peer review process. Furthermore, post-publication peer review raised concerns about the validity of the methods and statistical analysis, therefore the Editors no longer have confidence in the soundness of the findings. We apologise to all affected parties for the inconvenience caused.[41]

The film did not mention that Hooker's study has been retracted. If it had, there wouldn't have been a story to tell. Instead, the film blew Hooker's findings out of proportion, which is like raising your voice if you are short of arguments. Hooker said that the risk for African Americans to get a diagnosis of autism after vaccination was "astronomical" and highly statistically significant and that it was 8 on the Richter scale for earthquakes. No understatements here.

I tried my best to follow the arguments in the film that led to the conclusion that the CDC researchers had committed fraud, but there were no sound arguments. *Vaxxed* asked: Did the CDC commit fraud? The film tries to convince the viewers that it did, with four so-called exhibits, like in a court case: deviation from the analysis plan; omission of data; destruction of documents; and obstruction of justice. Let's take these claims one by one.

Wakefield said that the researchers deviated from their analysis plan when confronted with the risk in African Americans, and he also criticized that they used data on race not from the school records but from the birth certificates, which only half of the children had because the others were born in another state. The researchers reported that this allowed them to obtain additional information, such as birth weight and gestational age and the mother's parity, age, race, and education.[42]

Were data omitted and was this a problem? No. The film tuned in on the age groups, and there was a table, apparently from Thompson's internal report, that showed results for six rather narrow age groups separately, whereas the published paper operated with three age groups. I cannot see that this would make any difference to the results, and the three chosen age groups in the paper were highly reasonable, given the study's hypothesis. Researchers collapse groups all the time for clarity. The film showed what was called "handwritten notes" by Coleen Boyle from the CDC, something about reformatting and collapsing 19–23 with 24–35 months. Wakefield said that she tried new age groups, 0–11, 12–18, and 19–36 months, but that this failed, so in the end they dismissed the data altogether. Wakefield's criticism is inappropriate. The researchers showed their results using these age groups and explained why: less than 18 months was an indicator of "on-time" vaccination according to the recommended vaccination schedule; less than 24 months was the age range by which atypical development has become apparent in most children with autism; and less than 36 months defines the age by which autistic characteristics must have developed to meet DSM-IV criteria for autism.

Were documents destroyed? According to Hooker they were, because they showed a very strong statistically significant effect, and only Thompson retained them and gave them to Hooker, who filed an apparently groundless complaint with the Office of Research Integrity. According to the film, all people involved other than Thompson denied that there was a meeting where the documents were destroyed, and they called him a liar.

Thomson was scheduled to present the results of the CDC study, and he announced that he would say there was a causal association. The first author of the report, DeStefano, took over, and, according to the film, he reported falsely to the Institute of Medicine that there was no association. I must say I have sympathy with the CDC decision not to let Thompson present the results, as the study did not find any causal association. It even seems that Thompson accepted this conclusion because he coauthored the CDC paper.[43]

More than a decade later, Thompson delivered all the documents to Republican congressman Bill Posey, who commented on them in Congress on July 29, 2015. He recommended a thorough investigation be carried out and asked Congress to subpoena Thompson because he might face jail time if he spoke up without being subpoenaed. Wakefield lamented that, seven months later, Congress had done nothing. I fully understand why. There is nothing to be found.

Was there obstruction of justice? No. The film claimed that the CDC's fraudulent study had been used to deny the claims that children got autism from the vaccine. But there is no basis for such claims.

The film is highly manipulative in a multitude of other ways. A young boy had been instructed to say that isolated autism is a big problem because all healthy children are at risk. Using the same logic, flying is a big problem because we are all at risk for going down with the plane. He says that his sister is 18 months old, supposed to get the MMR vaccine, and that it is seven times more likely she will get autism than if the parents wait until she has become three years old. Bigtree refers to the CDC data as evidence for the "up to seven times" increased risk. But the children were white, not African American! And the confidence intervals were so wide that Bigtree might as well have said "down to almost no increased risk."[44] As a child, I once won a prize worth 200 Danish crowns for a photo I took with the shutter speed at 1/250 second. So, I could say: "Already as a child, I earned a lot of money, up to 180 million Danish crowns per hour." I could also say that I earned 2 crowns per hour by picking strawberries.

The film shows many heart-breaking interviews with parents who believe that vaccines made their child autistic, interspersed with home video footage of their low-functioning autistic children contrasted with earlier videos showing the same children looking happy and normal before the vaccination. At times, the parents tear up as they tell their story, which is a plea to make viewers believe the anecdotal evidence over the science.[45] I feel for these parents, of course, and I am not against using strongly emotive film sequences to convince people that they need to act, but only if the premises are correct, which they are not in this case.

The film's characters are carefully selected to compose the false narrative. Luc Montagnier won the Nobel Prize for the discovery of the virus that causes AIDS, and the film shows bits of the ceremony in Stockholm. In the film, Montagnier supports the autism theory, mentions that autism is more prominent in African Americans, and says that "this fraud, of course, ranks very high."

A specialist in autism, Doreen Granpeesheh, talks about its causes and mentions a so-called inability to detoxify what you are supposed to detoxify (which is language normally only used by quacks). The poisons come from vaccines, GMO products (I don't think there are any toxic problems with these), and the pesticides in our food (no relation to autism has ever been documented). Worst of all, she compares the 2014 Disneyland outbreak of 644 cases of measles with the number of autism cases, listed as 1,082,353.

The parents in the film are also carefully selected. Polly Tommey has an autistic son whose autism she blames on the MMR vaccine. She is the editor of *Autism File Magazine*, which peddles anti-vaccine pseudoscience and quack treatments for autism,[46] and she describes her mother as a "homeopathic hippie." She has worked closely with Wakefield on the Autism Media Channel.

I have observed that many people who are against vaccines are wedded to alternative medicine, even though none of it works.[47] If it did, doctors would no longer call it alternative medicine but simply use it.

Much of the movie features Wakefield repeating the same lies he's been repeating for two decades about how he came to want to investigate vaccines and autism, with no mention of his acceptance of large sums of money from a barrister looking to sue vaccine manufacturers. He sends the clear message that the "CDC whistleblower" vindicates him and recounts how he recommended the monovalent measles vaccine instead of the trivalent MMR, neglecting to mention his patent on this vaccine.

The movie doesn't mention Brian Deer, whose articles left Wakefield stark naked, as in "The Emperor's New Clothes."

Wakefield directed the film and says this about it on its homepage:

> For the last 20 years I have had to watch the suffering of those affected by autism as the problem multiplies year on year. What started with hope for a new understanding, new and effective treatments, and even prevention, turned to despair as special interests exploited their influence over the media to crush the science and the scientists.

Quite a remark considering that the special interests that distorted the whole thing were his own. And he continues:

> And then, two decades and a million damaged children later, one man, Dr. William Thompson—a CDC insider—decided to tell the truth and the embers of that early hope glow once more. Several years ago, I decided that to take on the media you had to become the media. The best medium for this story is film. Our aim with this movie was to take this complex, high-level fraud and to give it context, and weave through it the tragic street-level narratives of ordinary families affected by autism. This film brings to the public a dark and uncomfortable truth. To ignore it would be most unwise.

Wakefield doesn't see the irony. The complex, high-level fraud is his own, and the film brings to the public not a dark and uncomfortable truth, but a dark and uncomfortable lie.

The film was withdrawn from New York's 2016 Tribeca Film Festival after a public outcry.[48] Festival cofounder Robert de Niro, who has a child with autism, had bypassed the selection process in order to get *Vaxxed* a showing there. He needed to reverse his decision, which Wakefield called an act of censorship.

* * *

In 2018, *The Guardian* noted that Wakefield, under the anti-establishment presidency of Donald Trump, had become a leading light in the United States and frighteningly influential worldwide.[49] Wakefield and his supporters insist mainstream science is wrong and will not be persuaded otherwise. The conspiracy theories of the anti-vax movement, which *Vaxxed* exemplifies, are all over the Internet, and the apparent acceptance of Wakefield into the upper echelons of American society can only boost them further.

This reminds me of a famous Danish businessman who said it doesn't matter if you get bad press; it is better than no press.

Wakefield is the prime reason why many parents refuse having their children vaccinated and spew every kind of concern, not only about MMR, but over vaccinations in general, which have had disastrous consequences for some of them.

In America, a ferocious anti-vaccine movement took off after Wakefield toured US autism conferences and after he, in November 2000, appeared on the CBS Network's *60 Minutes* linking MMR with what he called an epidemic of autism. This was followed by campaigners' claims that all vaccines are suspect.

Wakefield's false claims provide a foundation for continued fundraising from parents of autistic children, many of whom have been led to believe that Wakefield is their champion.

Alliance for Human Research Protection Calls Wakefield a Hero

In 2016, when I asked to have my name removed from the Alliance's website, https://ahrp.org/, the bio for Wakefield was 2 pages. When I checked it in 2019, it was 12 pages. In both versions, Wakefield is quoted as saying: "I was not responsible for their clinical care—that was performed by an outstanding group of gastroenterologists who confirmed, beyond a shadow of a doubt, that these children have an inflammatory bowel disease and that has now been replicated around the world."

None of Wakefield's 12 children in the *Lancet* paper had inflammatory bowel disease, and it has not been replicated. The bio is full of other grave errors, derogatory comments, colorful adjectives, and conspiracy postulates, typical for vaccine deniers. It is also a smear campaign against Brian Deer, and it sanctifies Wakefield.

Wakefield's "notoriety" is said to have been generated by a relentless series of sensationalist articles and reignited by the editor-in-chief of the *BMJ*: "The *BMJ* embarked on a smear campaign calculated to cause the greatest damage to Dr. Wakefield." I wonder how Vera Sharav, the president of the Alliance, can know which motives people have?

In the most recent version of Wakefield's bio, this sentence had been removed: "A concerted effort has been to divert attention from regulatory failure to protect children. Instead, mainstream media has followed Brian Deer's attack-dog tactics and conducted a relentless crusade to destroy Dr. Wakefield's reputation and character." Wakefield destroyed himself by his dishonesty; no conspiracy (concerted effort), crusade, or dog fight was needed for this.

This is also not true: "The parents of the children in the *Lancet* study sought Dr. Wakefield's help for their children, based on his previous publications." Sharav does not mention anything about Wakefield's involvement with the planned litigation being the incentive for fishing for these parents.

"The case against Andrew Wakefield is driven by corporations whose financial interests collide with independent medical investigations that identify troublesome safety issues." It wasn't. It was one courageous man's work: Brian Deer. In 2011, Deer was named specialist journalist of the year in the British newspaper industry's annual Pulitzer-style press awards. Judges for the Society of Editors praised his "outstanding perseverance, stamina and revelation on a story of major importance."[50]

Sharav writes about a culture of intimidation, which the pharmaceutical industry has subjected Wakefield to, but the drug industry had nothing to do with Wakefield's self-inflicted demise, and the intimidation was the other way around. Wakefield launched frivolous lawsuits against Deer. Sharav says nothing about this, and we are supposed to pity the villain: "Wakefield has been vilified and subjected to false accusations orchestrated by the interconnected shadows who control the dissemination of medical information. They were determined to destroy his reputation, his credibility, his professional integrity and his career."

Wakefield's assertion about the measles vaccine being the cause of his new syndrome, autistic enterocolitis, has never been replicated by others, but Sharav writes: Read our compilation of "Scientific reports validate 'controversial findings reported in *The Lancet.*'"

Sharav mentions that Thomas Verstraeten assessed the risk of thimerosal, the mercury preservative in some vaccines, using a large US database, and found that exposure to thimerosal during the first month of life increased the relative risk of autism by 7.6%. She misrepresents an abstract from 1999 that noted that the risk ratio was 7.6 (1.8 to 31.5).[51] Thus, the risk was increased 7.6 times, which is far more than 7.6%, but the result is highly uncertain, as indicated by the wide confidence interval. Furthermore, register studies are bias prone, and results published only in abstracts are often misleading. I could not find any publication of Verstraeten's study, but he published another large database study in 2003.[52] In this study, the positive findings were so small that they should be ignored. There was an increased risk of tics, risk ratio 1.89 (1.05 to 3.38), and language delay, risk ratio 1.13 (1.01 to 1.27). None of the analyses found significantly increased risks for autism or attention-deficit disorder. Verstraeten concluded that no consistent associations were found between thimerosal-containing vaccines and neurodevelopmental outcomes.

Sharav does not mention this study, but three studies that did not find any link between thimerosal-containing vaccines and autism.[53] She dismisses them with the claim that others have shown that these influential studies are fraudulent. If claiming that important studies are fraudulent, one must always give the references, but Sharav keeps her readers in total darkness.

The three studies were published in prestigious journals: *New England Journal of Medicine*,[54] *Pediatrics*,[55] and *Journal of the American Medical Association (JAMA)*.[56] All were from Denmark. We are world famous for our meticulous register studies, and we have some of the best registers in the world. All three studies are highly convincing, and as they are very large, it is not likely they overlooked anything.

In the first study, from 2002, 82% of 537,303 children in the cohort had received the MMR vaccine.[57] The authors identified 316 children with autism and 422 with autism spectrum disorders. After adjustment for potential confounders, the risk ratio for autism among vaccinated children, as compared with the unvaccinated ones, was 0.92 (0.68 to 1.24), and the risk ratio for autistic spectrum disorder was 0.83 (0.65 to 1.07). There was no association between the age at time of vaccination, the time since vaccination, or the date of vaccination and the development of autistic disorder. The authors concluded that their study provides strong evidence against the hypothesis that MMR vaccination causes autism. I agree. It is a very strong study, which the CDC researchers also concluded was much stronger than their own study,[58] and yet Del Bigtree and Andrew Wakefield made a whole film about the CDC study and ignored the Danish one!

The second study included 956 children diagnosed with autism during 1971–2000.[59] There was no increase in the incidence of autism during the period when thimerosal was used in Denmark, until 1990. From 1991, the incidence increased, but also among children born *after* the discontinuation of thimerosal.

In the third study, of a cohort of 467,450 children, the researchers compared those vaccinated with a thimerosal-containing vaccine with those vaccinated with another formulation of the same vaccine.[60] There were 440 autism cases and 787 cases of other autism spectrum disorders. The risk was similar for the two groups, risk ratio 0.85 (0.60 to 1.20) for autism and 1.12 (0.88 to 1.43) for other autism spectrum disorders. Furthermore, there was no dose-response relationship: The increase in risk ratio per 25 µg of ethylmercury was nonexistent, namely, 0.98 (0.90 to 1.06) for autism and 1.03 (0.98 for 1.09) for other autism spectrum disorders.

Sharav does not say a word about these three highly convincing studies apart from postulating with no evidence that they are fraudulent. Instead, she tells us Dr. Wakefield has harmed no child whereas the medical journals and the media turn a blind eye to the catastrophic harms that hundreds of thousands of children and their families experience.

Sharav briefly mentions William Thompson's "whistleblowing" and says that the data concealed a fourfold increased rate of autism in black baby boys. Sharav goes on and on like this. The GMC trial against Wakefield she calls a "kangaroo court," and her views are that the case was concocted, that he had no conflicts of interest, and that he is an honest scientist.

Deer's ground-breaking research she calls a "flame-throwing style of irresponsible journalism," and BMJ's editorial[61] is "defamatory." But facts cannot be defamatory. It is a fact that Wakefield falsified the data.

Sharav writes that the British High Court overturned the GMC panel's verdict and exonerated one of Wakefield's coauthors, John Walker-Smith, who had appealed the GMC's action. Wakefield apologists abuse this verdict to also exonerate Wakefield, but the judgment had nothing to do with him. According to Deer, Walker-Smith and Wakefield were both financially supported by the Medical Protection Society, which had agreed to Walker-Smith appealing, but rejected Wakefield, on advice from his own legal team. Had he appealed, the GMC would have reconvened the panel and most likely struck him off again from the license to practice register. That was their right, and they could have done it to Walker-Smith but didn't, because he was about 73, and to prolong the nightmare Wakefield had put him through might have seriously impacted his health.

Sharav claims that the High Court decision invalidates the GMC process and its charge of fraud against Wakefield and that there was no fraud in the Lancet study. It is unbelievable how manipulative she is. In her letter to me, she wrote that the GMC proceedings had been discredited. They have not. They are valid, and all the material was gathered by the GMC's own lawyers.

Sharav writes that BMJ's accusation of fraud was itself a fabrication and that the mudslinging would never stand up in a court of law. Of course it would, and the *BMJ* editors asserted that there was clear evidence of falsification.[62]

Sharav asserts that others have replicated Wakefield's findings. She offers a hyperlink that doesn't work, and I couldn't find the material in a Google search, so I assume it has been removed, if it ever existed. *BMJ* and I are not aware of any confirmatory studies. Apart from this, there will always be many highly flawed papers that purport to have shown something that supports popular beliefs, so it is not a matter of whether some odd papers like the retracted study by Hooker exist, but it is a matter of whether there is any *reliable* research. The hypothesis about the measles vaccine causing autism should be relegated to the graveyard of discredited medical hypotheses, if there is any room left.

Sharav ends her sanctification of Wakefield with an amusing remark: "Even a cursory examination of the scientific reports validating Dr. Wakefield's controversial findings, convinces us of the scientific integrity of the much disparaged article. We have, therefore, concluded that Dr. Andrew Wakefield is indeed a hero for his courageous stand."

A cursory examination cannot validate Wakefield's findings unless it is done with the eyes closed. The vaccine deniers ignore the indisputable scientific evidence that Wakefield's research is fraudulent[63] and depict Wakefield as being the victim of a societal conspiracy that forced him to leave England and go to the United States. I say indisputable because it *is* indisputable. It is very rare that anything is indisputable in science, but in this case it is. The evidence of fraud is so stunning in every detail that it cannot be questioned.

Wakefield's so-called bio has no authors. I supposed it was written by Sharav even though it says that "we" concluded Wakefield is a hero. I asked Sharav and the Board of Directors about it, and it turned out that only Sharav has concluded Wakefield is a hero.

Public Statements by Physicians for Informed Consent (PIC)

Shira Miller, a physician, founded Physicians for Informed Consent (PIC) in 2015, after the mandatory vaccination law (SB277) for school attendance passed in California. It is an educational, nonprofit organization whose mission is to safeguard informed consent (and informed refusal) in vaccination. Miller wrote to me that the volunteer leadership of PIC is comprised of physicians, scientists, and attorneys and that their membership includes thousands of patients, the general public, and a coalition of over 100 international organizations. As already noted, when she invited me to speak at her meeting in March 2019, she encouraged me to criticize what she had written about measles, which I shall do now.

Miller wrote in *BMJ*[64] that "our organization has found that it has not been proven that the MMR vaccine results in less death or permanent disability than what is expected from measles."[65] She argued that the risk of dying or suffering permanent injury from measles in the United States was very small, even before the measles vaccine was introduced in 1963, and that the risk of dying from measles before vaccination was only 1 in 10,000 or 0.01%.[66] She asserted that the official risk of 1 in 1,000, e.g., from the CDC, is that high because only 10% of measles cases are reported.

Miller quoted a large Danish study that reported 1.56 MMR-related febrile seizure cases per 1,000 vaccinated children aged 15 to 17 months within 2 weeks of the vaccination.[67] The researchers described this risk difference to unvaccinated children as small. It was also transient (after 2 weeks the risk was even a little lower in the vaccinated than in the unvaccinated group). Some perspective is clearly needed. Although 82% of the children were vaccinated, only 5% (973) of the seizures occurred within 2 weeks of the vaccination. Thus, instead of 973, there would have been 624 seizures without vaccination (973/1.56). This means that only 2% (349/17,986) of the febrile seizures were caused by vaccination, and this did not lead to more cases of epilepsy. It is therefore a trivial harm, particularly if compared to the beneficial effects of the vaccine on mortality and morbidity.

Miller wrote that the risk of febrile seizures after MMR vaccination, 1 in 640,[68] is fivefold higher than the risk from measles, but the data she compared are not comparable. First, the Danish registries are far more complete than US registries, and the data she used for the comparison came from the CDC,[69] which she had just criticized for 90% underreporting. Second, Miller's estimate is indirect and highly uncertain. She argued that measles surveillance had shown 3 to 3.5 times more measles seizures than measles deaths,[70] and she then used her own low measles case-fatality rate of one 1 in 10,000 to calculate a seizure rate from measles of 1 in 3,100. Third, seizure risk after vaccination should not be compared to seizure risk after measles. What should be compared is total mortality and morbidity (not only including seizures, but also, for example, permanent brain damage), and if this is done, there is no doubt that vaccination wins by far, and that the difference in seizures is trivial.

PIC's information leaflet about the MMR vaccine is also problematic.[71] Miller quotes CDC when saying that serious allergic reactions occur once per one million doses: "However, other severe side effects include deafness, long-term seizures, coma, lowered consciousness, permanent brain damage, and death. While the CDC states that these side effects are rare, the precise numbers are unknown." Such information is seriously misleading and looks like a scare campaign. As MMR is an attenuated live virus vaccine, it may cause similar problems as infections with measles, mumps, and rubella, but the infections are far worse than the vaccines. Millions of people would die and many more would be harmed if we did not vaccinate.

She says, "Additionally, the manufacturer's package insert states, 'M-M-R II vaccine has not been evaluated for carcinogenic or mutagenic potential, or potential to impair fertility.'" This is also seriously misleading. What about the potential for the infections to cause such harms? For example, rubella may cause miscarriage, preterm birth, or stillbirth, as well as a variety of birth defects, but Miller says nothing about such issues.

A figure in the leaflet shows that the risk of permanent injury from the MMR vaccine is 4 times higher than the risk of dying from measles in the United States.[72] However, it is obscure how Miller derived the risk of permanent injury, 4 in 10,000, or what the injury is. This risk is unbelievably high. It is 32 times larger than Miller's estimate for permanent injury after measles in the same leaflet, 1 in 80,000, which cannot be correct. Miller quotes another of her leaflets for this low disease risk, and it turns out that injury means permanent disability from measles encephalitis, i.e., brain damage. Well, according to Miller herself, 1 in 10,000 die due to measles (in reality, it is at least 10 in 10,000 who die, which I shall discuss soon). Is it not "permanent disability" to be dead, which should therefore have been included?

Miller's estimates are invalid, and she compares apples and oranges. The worst blunder is that the reason that so few people die is that almost the whole population is vaccinated!

Miller criticizes one of the large Danish studies, the one from *New England Journal of Medicine*,[73] but her discussion of this study is uninterpretable. She notes that there was a difference between the data adjusted for confounders (reported in the paper) and the raw data (which were not reported). She did not explain where she got the raw data from and what they showed, and it escapes me how she could claim that the study did not rule out the possibility that the MMR vaccine increases the risk of an adverse event that leads to permanent injury by up to 77%. She might equally well have said that the study did not rule out the possibility that the vaccine decreased the risk of an adverse event by some amount. In fact, the vaccine *does* decrease the risk of permanent injury quite substantially. But vaccine deniers are not interested in the truth. When they see it, they distort it beyond recognition.

Why Are Measles Vaccines Important?

According to WHO, there were 110,000 measles deaths in 2017, and most were in children under the age of five.[74] Vaccination resulted in an 80% drop in measles deaths between 2000 and 2017, preventing an estimated 21 million deaths. Before the vaccine was introduced in 1963, major epidemics occurred causing an estimated 2.6 million deaths each year. The most serious complications to measles include blindness, encephalitis (an infection that causes brain swelling), severe diarrhea and dehydration, ear infections, and severe respiratory infections such as bacterial pneumonia.

WHO did not mention that the vaccine also protects against the increased risk of dying from other infections. A study in *Science* from 2015 reported that the risk of dying from other infections after a measles infection is increased during the next 2–3 years.[75] The authors explained that this is because measles cause immunosuppression, likely via depletion of B and T lymphocytes. However, it seems that the investigators cherry-picked their data,[76] and at any rate, their hypothesis cannot explain Aaby's finding that vaccination against measles decreases total mortality much more than predicted by its specific effect against measles even in settings where no one got measles.[77] Thus, it seems likely that the measles vaccine has beneficial immune training effects and measles itself may also have such effects. The investigators confirmed Aaby's finding that the nonspecific benefits of vaccination are stronger in females than in males.

It is important to avoid getting infected because there are no antiviral treatments for measles. WHO recommends that all children with measles should receive two doses of vitamin A, given 24 hours apart, to prevent blindness and other eye damage and because it reduces the number of deaths from measles by 50%.[78]

Is this correct? A Google search on *vitamin A Cochrane measles* finds the relevant Cochrane review:

> After a single dose, there was no significant reduction in mortality in the vitamin A group, risk ratio 0.70 (0.42 to 1.15). However, two doses of vitamin A (200,000 international units on consecutive days) reduced the mortality in children aged less than two years, risk ratio 0.21 (0.07 to 0.66).[79]

We should always check the evidence behind official recommendations. Although I do not doubt that measles vaccines save millions of lives, I asked WHO what their evidence was for the numbers of lives saved.[80] It was not easy to find out whom to contact because the report had no authors. On WHO's website, where I found the report, I went from *Who We Are* to *Contact Us*, where I found an envelope, which usually means that one can submit questions via this route, but the link was dead. I was unable to find an email address I could use. There was a phone number, but I don't use the phone when I have questions about science; I need a written reply. In such situations, I often use the media option. There was something called *For General Inquiries*, but it sent me back to the page I came from, with the phone number!

I was about to give up when I found an email to be used if the matter is urgent: mediainquiries@who.int. So, I needed to pretend I was a journalist and that my matter was urgent. This is a common problem with big organizations. It is usually impossible to write to a drug company's headquarters. There is no email address anywhere. Some organizations seem not to want to be contacted by anyone.

In my email, I suggested that WHO link to the evidence, which is needed if WHO wanted to be an evidence-based organization, so that researchers can check it: "Can you please send my suggestion to the relevant office, copying me, so that I can see the email address?"

I didn't get a reply from WHO's press office, so I sent a reminder, which didn't help, either.

It is easy to look up the relevant Cochrane review of the MMR vaccine by googling *measles Cochrane*.[81] The authors included five randomized trials, one controlled clinical trial, 27 cohort studies, 17 case-control studies, five time-series trials, one case cross-over trial, two ecological studies, and six self-controlled case series studies, involving a total of about 15 million people.

One MMR vaccine dose reduced the risk of measles by 95% and the risk of secondary cases among household contacts by 92%. The risk of febrile seizures was slightly increased in one large cohort study involving half a million children, risk ratio 1.10 (1.05 to 1.15) and somewhat more in other studies, relative incidence 4.09 (3.10 to 5.33) and 5.68 (2.31 to 13.97). The risk of thrombocytopenic purpura was increased in a case-control study, odds ratio 6.3 (1.3 to 30.1).

No relation was found between the MMR vaccine and autism, asthma, leukemia, hay fever, Type I diabetes, gait disturbance, Crohn's disease,

demyelinating diseases, and bacterial or viral infections. The authors concluded that the design and reporting of safety outcomes in the reviewed
studies were largely inadequate.

People who are concerned about the rising rates of autism and think it
is caused by vaccines are barking up the wrong tree. If autism is caused by
some external factor, it would be far more relevant to investigate the effect of
brain-active substances like depression pills when given to pregnant women
or to pregnant experimental animals.

There were no data on deaths in the studies in the Cochrane review.
However, when the vaccine is highly effective in preventing measles, it would
be expected to be also highly effective in reducing mortality. Observational
data on measles incidence and mortality are very convincing, and I show
below a graph from the CDC, which is slightly inaccurate; the introduction
of the vaccine occurred in 1963, a little earlier than the arrow shows[82]:

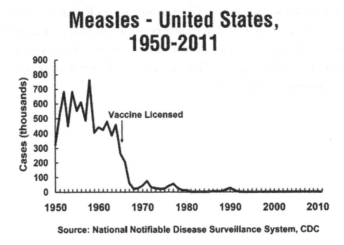

Source: National Notifiable Disease Surveillance System, CDC

Measles outbreaks also provide strong support for the benefits of the vaccine. In the United States, there was a resurgence of measles in 1989–1990,
which primarily involved unvaccinated racial and ethnic minority children
less than five years of age residing in inner-city areas.[83] There were 66 (0.1%)
cases of encephalitis. A provisional total of 41 measles-associated deaths was
reported in 1989 (2.3 deaths per 1000 cases), which increased to 89 (3.2 per
1000 cases) in 1990.

In 2000, the CDC declared measles eradicated in the United States, but
there have been several outbreaks since due to imported cases.[84] In 2018, no
fewer than 17 outbreaks occurred. One, in New York, was due to people

who had been to Israel, and it included 182 cases in orthodox Jewish communities with a vaccination rate of only 50%.[85]

It is not possible to say exactly what the risk is of dying from measles. As noted earlier, the death risk is related to the infectious dose, which is higher in settings with overcrowding. We can only say what it has been in outbreaks, and a commonly used estimate is 2 deaths per 1000 cases. But it can be much worse. During an epidemic in Copenhagen in 1887, at least 5% of the children, or 50 per 1000 cases, died.[86] The mortality was probably even higher because only those who died while they had a rash counted. In Vienna, at the beginning of the twentieth century, the mortality was 11% among the poorest and 0.6% among the richest.

An outbreak in Madagascar that started in 2018 had, in April 2019, caused over 1200 deaths, which is about 1% of those infected.[87] Only about 60% of the population is vaccinated.

We should all get vaccinated against measles and get our children vaccinated, with very few exceptions. Contraindications for the vaccine include a history of severe allergic reaction to any component of the vaccine including neomycin, pregnancy (measles illness during pregnancy results in a higher risk of premature labor, spontaneous abortion, and low-birthweight infants), and severe immunosuppression.[88]

3

Mandatory Vaccinations?

As a prelude to this chapter, events in Japan are interesting. Japan stopped using the MMR vaccine in 1993 after many children had developed meningitis and other adverse reactions.[1] There had been three deaths, while eight children were left with permanent handicaps ranging from damaged hearing and blindness to loss of control of limbs. Japan had used a type of MMR that included a particular strain of mumps vaccine that was later discontinued because of safety concerns (see Chapter 8).

The Japanese government realized there was a problem with the MMR they were using soon after its introduction in April 1989, when vaccination was compulsory. Parents who refused to have their child vaccinated needed to pay a small fine. One in every 900 children was experiencing problems of various kinds, which was over 2,000 times the expected rate.

In 1993, after a public outcry fueled by worries over the flu vaccine, the Japanese government dropped the requirement for children to be vaccinated and started using the vaccines one by one rather than in combination. But it came with a cost. Although this happened many years ago, it led to lower vaccination rates, and measles outbreaks occurred, which took 94 lives in the last five years up to 2019.[2]

The Japanese experience tells us that vaccinations are a delicate issue, and that it is easy to go from bad to worse when the public make far-reaching decisions based on rare harms. Vaccines are generally very safe, and a few deaths should not lead to anti-vaccination sentiments. It is also very safe to travel by air, much safer than ground travel, but people react differently. Even though plane crashes have killed thousands of people, we continue to travel by air. I therefore cannot understand why the same people do not accept that, very rarely, something goes wrong with vaccines, which should not influence our decision making.

But it surely does, even when the harm concerns a totally different vaccine. On February 14, 2019, the *BMJ* reported that 70 people, most of them children, had died of measles in the Philippines since the start of 2019, i.e., in less than two months.[3] There were over 18,000 cases of measles in 2018, compared to only about 2,400 the year before. Measles vaccination rates fell from a high of 88% in 2014 to about 55% in 2018. This was caused by a political battle over Sanofi's dengue vaccine, Dengvaxia, which was discontinued in the Philippines in 2018 after several deaths had occurred in vaccinated children (see Chapter 9).

Given such experiences with citizens who are not reacting rationally, I can understand why some authorities have made vaccination against certain viruses mandatory, or why they ban access to school for children who are not vaccinated against measles. Sometimes, drastic measures are needed to protect the population. In the Middle Ages, weeks of quarantine were mandatory for the crew on ships that arrived from Asia at Italian ports to protect the population against plague, which, in the worst epidemics, killed one-third of the population. People were scared to death, and plague was called the Black Death because of the bleeding it causes, which leads to black encrustations.

Drastic measures may have some effect. State closure of the nonmedical exemption, based on religious or philosophical beliefs, in some US states has resulted in increased coverage of the MMR vaccine.[4]

However, we should discuss whether such drastic measures are defensible when we don't face anything remotely as threatening as plague. In California, a school or other institution may require documentary proof of each entrant's immunization status according to the law. The required immunizations are against diphtheria, hepatitis B, Haemophilus influenzae type b, measles, mumps, pertussis (whooping cough), poliomyelitis, rubella, tetanus, varicella (chicken pox), and any other disease deemed appropriate by the department.

In 2015, the exemption based upon personal beliefs was removed.[5] In the first year after the change was implemented, the percentage of kindergartners entering school not up to date on vaccinations decreased from 7.2% to 4.4%.[6]

In the worst case, mandatory vaccinations might lead to disasters if it turns out that a particular vaccine, or combination of vaccines, has led to serious harm.

The recommended vaccinations in the United States have reduced the incidence of several infectious diseases by over 99%, e.g., measles, mumps and rubella,[7] and some are considered eradicated, e.g., diphtheria, polio, and smallpox.[8] It has been estimated that for a single birth cohort, nearly 20 million cases of diseases and over 40,000 deaths are prevented. Another analysis showed that an investment in 10 vaccines in 94 low- and middle-income countries resulted in savings almost 50 times as large when broader economic benefits were included.

Countries vary a lot in the ideals they treasure. I doubt that drastic measures like mandatory vaccinations would ever see the light of day again in my country, Denmark (we have had it for smallpox, from 1810 to 1976). We value our individual freedom far too much for that to happen, but the Unites States is a very different country. Religious fundamentalism is much more common than in other Western nations, with weird ideas and rules about what to do and what not and irrational beliefs that go totally against the most reliable scientific knowledge we have.

Here is a concrete example. What should we do with parents like the ones who did not ensure that their 6-year-old boy became vaccinated against tetanus, and whose tetanus cost nearly $1 million of care?[9] He cut his forehead while playing outdoors on a farm. After 57 days in an Oregon pediatric acute care unit, the parents refused the recommended second dose of tetanus vaccine. The recommendation is five doses during childhood and a booster shot every ten years throughout life. The pediatrician said: "I've seen close to 100 patients who needed intensive care because of a disease that is preventable by vaccine. I've never had to give intensive care because of complications from a vaccine."

I can understand why US authorities feel they need to introduce drastic measures when too many people are out of reach for rational arguments and when powerful lobby groups escalate the problem by spreading lethal misinformation about vaccines on the Internet. In Denmark, I have never heard about any anti-vaxxer movement, and Wakefield's name is never mentioned. We ignore him. The media are also far more critical toward fake news than in the United States, which means that any attempt at mendacious scaremongering in relation to the harms of vaccines would be quickly exposed for what it is.

But it seems that the United States is not so special after all. We also have mandatory vaccinations in Europe. When I searched for it on Google, I found a website sponsored by multiple vaccine manufacturers, *VaccinesToday*. I always check the *About Us* section on websites and would not normally read anything from a drug company-sponsored website but made an exception, as I came across an article from 2017 that seemed okay and factual.[10] Furthermore, it concluded that the benefits of mandatory vaccination are questionable, which is not in the sponsors' interest, so I read on. Compulsory vaccination was first introduced in the United Kingdom through the 1853 Vaccination Act. The law required that all children—whose health permits—be vaccinated against smallpox and obliged physicians to certify that vaccination had taken place. Parents who refused could be fined £1 (about £130 today).

Today, no vaccines are currently mandated in the United Kingdom,[11] and public health leaders have long resisted compulsory vaccination on the grounds that it undermines the trust between the public and healthcare professionals. It is seen as counterproductive, but there is now a renewed push for mandates in the United Kingdom,[12] which has increasingly come to resemble the United States rather than other European countries.[13] The lack of personal freedom is also similar. Staff members in the National Health Service who refuse to have the flu vaccine will need to provide their employer with their reasons.[14] Its national director said, "we all have a professional responsibility to protect ourselves and, by doing so, better protect our patients and reducing the pressure on services." This is the typical nonsense we constantly see from those at the top. It is also nonevidence-based (see next chapter) and violates fundamental human rights. What on Earth is happening? Surely, healthcare workers have an ethical imperative to prevent harm to patients, but this imperative has been abused as an argument in favor of mandatory vaccination.[15] The counterargument wins: compulsion strips healthcare providers of a basic right guaranteed to every other patient—the right to informed consent.[16]

I believe it is impossible to argue rationally for mandatory vaccination of healthcare workers with flu shots to protect the patients against some theoretical risk that they might contract influenza. It is an intrusion in one person's body in order to *possibly* (this hasn't even been documented in reliable research) lower the risk of something untoward happening to another person. I cannot recall any other instance in society where we ask one person to provide a sacrifice for the possible benefit of another, apart from war times, not to mention *mandating* it. No vaccine is entirely harmless, and in the worst case, the healthcare worker might die, e.g., because of an anaphylactic shock caused by the vaccine, or fainting with head trauma after the injection, or development of Guillain-Barré syndrome, all of which can be deadly.

In this book, I have exposed the horrific wrongs committed by vaccine deniers, but there are also huge problems on the other side. Some fundamentalists can only see positive consequences of vaccinations. When such people are in power, things can go badly wrong. In 2017, a senior faculty member at the New York University School of Medicine, who did not even do clinical work, had her faculty appointment terminated because she did not get an influenza vaccination.[17] The university stated that "immunization against the flu is critical for the protection of our patients, visitors, and colleagues. Regrettably, since we have not received evidence of your vaccination, your non-compensated faculty appointment will be terminated effective immediately."

It is no wonder that some people speak about health fascism when the do-gooders seem to have no limits to their violations of basic human rights. Another example from New York illustrates that we should not give up the fight. A lawyer successfully struck down as illegal the New York City Department of Health's flu shot requirement for preschoolers.[18] This was a well-deserved victory for human rights. The requirement was unjustified, both ethically and scientifically (see next chapter). Unfortunately, the victory was overturned by the highest court.

* * *

In ethical discussions, the slippery slope argument plays an important role. It is related to the consistency principle and goes something like this: Although it may seem reasonable in this concrete case to do this, it could open the door to other things we would not like to accept but would be forced to accept because we would be unable to identify an ethically relevant difference between the two situations. It is much the same in law, and a related argument is: I might be tempted to cheat in this situation, but what if everyone else cheated in similar situations? Perhaps we would lose trust in one another, and our society would break down?

The examples from New York with the influenza vaccine illustrate the importance of the slippery slope argument. The required immunizations in California did not include influenza, but this could change because the law provided for any other disease deemed appropriate by the department. We should never give people, who already have a lot of power, even more power. History has taught us that it always goes wrong.

In New York State, a bill is under way prohibiting children to go to school unless vaccinated against HPV. But HPV does not spread in the classroom. There seems to be no limit to the insanity in public health. Or, do we just see the result of corruption?

Healthcare in Australia also has many similarities to that in the United States, so it is not surprising that in this country, compliance with child-hood immunization schedules has been linked to preschool admission and to family assistance payments ("No jab, no pay").[19]

In most instances where vaccine mandates are in force, they apply only to children. However, vaccination is linked to employment in some institu-tions—notably in healthcare facilities. This is not a legal mandate per se, but a form of discrimination. I have been informed by a UK colleague that, at some hospitals, if the employees get the flu and are not vaccinated, there will be no money for a substitute. A trade union representative working at a UK hospital that imposed mandatory flu vaccinations for staff had complained to the administration, but it was not upheld. His trade union supported him, but the staff had been threatened with disciplinary action for refusing to be vaccinated, and they had a clause in their contract of employment about this.

The uncertainties related to the scientific and ethical justifications for mandatory vaccination are reflected in the highly varying policies in Europe. A 2010 study of 27 EU countries (plus Iceland and Norway) found that 15 had no mandatory vaccines.[20] Since then, "Italy has added 10 vac-cines to its list of compulsory vaccines; France and Romania are preparing new laws that would penalise parents of unvaccinated children; and Finland will introduce legislation in March 2018 that requires health and social care providers to ensure staff are immunised against measles, varicella, pertussis and influenza."

In 2017, Robb Butler from WHO wrote a letter to the US Senate Health Commission. He noted that, based on a 2011 report, vaccination against polio was mandatory in 12 countries in western Europe, diphtheria and teta-nus in 11, and hepatitis B in 10. The WHO paper on measles vaccination recommends that children should be screened for measles vaccination at the time of school entry and that those who had not received two doses should be vaccinated; 12 countries required proof of vaccination at school entry.

Butler mentioned that, to mitigate the negative impact of misinforma-tion, it is vitally important to provide accurate and evidence-based infor-mation on the benefits and safety of vaccines. Further, we should listen carefully to the concerns of parents and the public in general and better meet their needs so that they can make informed choices for themselves and their children.

The impact of mandates in Europe has been assessed by the EU-funded ASSET project, which found no clear link to vaccine uptake. ASSET experts have also argued that while mandatory vaccination might fix a short-term problem, it is not a long-term solution. Better organization of healthcare systems and strong communication strategies may prove more effective. The EU commissioner with responsibility for health noted that "The legitimate goal of achieving the highest possible immunization rates can be attained through less stringent policies, and most Member States prefer the adoption of 'recommendation policies' or else a mix of obligation/recommendation policies."[21] A professor said that mandates do not improve vaccine confidence, but make opposition to vaccination even stronger.[22]

I agree. But as described in the previous chapter, I cancelled my talk in California opposing mandatory vaccination when I found out that the respectable title of the organization, Physicians for Informed Consent, was a veiled code term for being against vaccines as a "matter of principle," which is indisputably wrong. Moreover, one cannot talk about informed consent to refuse vaccination, e.g., for measles, when the parents have been terribly misinformed by doctors like Wakefield and his followers.

Principles for Ethical Argumentation

I have already mentioned the slippery slope argument and the requirement of consistency. When dealing with ethical dilemmas, it is not acceptable to let intuition and feelings about right and wrong guide decisions. "I think, I feel, I believe" are commonly heard but have no ethical value. There are rules that must be respected in a rational ethical debate.[23]

First, we need to get the facts right, just like in a court case. What does the science tell us?

Second, even when we agree on the facts, we cannot derive an "ought" from an "is," as the "ought" involves an ethical choice. We cannot derive "we must" from "we can."

Third, as already noted, there needs to be consistency. If two cases are treated differently, we must be able to demonstrate an ethically relevant difference between them. This principle is very often ignored in debates.

Fourth, we need to decide on whether we weigh the deontological perspective, which is about prima facie duties such as respecting people's autonomy, higher than the utilitarian perspective. Utilitarianism has to do with the consequences of our actions, and we strive for the greatest good for the greatest number. It is well known in the form of paternalism, which comes in three different forms:

Genuine paternalism, where, for example, parents care for their children, or doctors do their best to help comatose people survive;

Solicited paternalism, where, for example, the patient facing different choices asks the doctor to decide, or a guest at a restaurant gets confused about all the options and asks the waiter to choose something; and

Unsolicited paternalism, where the patient did not give permission for others to intervene, e.g., forced medication in psychiatry. It is often argued that psychotic patients cannot take care of themselves, but this argument is doubtful, as they can be fully rational when rejecting treatment with a neuroleptic because they know it is highly unpleasant and dangerous.[24]

Based on utilitarian reasoning, it can be argued that a person could be thrown overboard from a sinking boat if this helps the remaining people survive. This is where the principle of deontology becomes important. Deontology is about duties, irrespective of the consequences, and one of our duties is to not kill people. Therefore, when principles of utilitarianism and deontology clash, we normally behave like deontologists, but this is not the case in all cultures. In some cultures, the society is far more important than the individual. Deontology is also about our rights, and respect for autonomy and respect for the patient's dignity are examples.

One of the major problems in healthcare is the many busybodies who love telling others what they should do, even when no one asked them, and outright arrogance is also common, particularly when the patients have another view. The result of this unsolicited paternalism is all over the place, as if people were not trusted to think for themselves, e.g., the title for an official information leaflet might be "Why you should get screened for breast cancer" instead of "Should you get screened for breast cancer?"

Returning to vaccinations, should parents be allowed to refuse them for their children based on their erroneous beliefs? Let's try to use the consistency principle. In Denmark, an adult has the right to refuse a life-saving blood transfusion. People belonging to the Jehovah's Witnesses sect firmly refuse blood transfusions, and one such woman who was bleeding profusely after childbirth was told that she would very likely die if she refused transfusions. She refused, and she died. As she was fully conscious and knew the consequences of her choice, it was not allowed to transfuse her, not even if she had become unconscious. This may seem cruel, but her wish was respected, and she is not the only one who has died because of her religious beliefs.

But if a child of a Jehovah's Witness is brought in after a traffic accident and the parents refuse life-saving transfusions, the state is obliged to protect the vulnerable minor, just like in any other case of child neglect, and the child will get the transfusion.

We cannot compare this situation directly with that of parents who refuse to have their child vaccinated against measles because the child is not in immediate danger, but if it could be considered child neglect, the state might intervene.

We also have duties toward one another, and by refusing vaccinations, the parents increase the risk that their child—and themselves, as they made the decision—will harm other people.

Some people are free riders: "If I let the others run a very small risk of getting harmed by the vaccine, then I shall not get vaccinated because there will be herd immunity and I shall therefore not get infected." It is easy to see that this attitude is unethical. If everyone thought like you, we would all be bad off. The opposite of having a kind of parasitic relationship with fellow human beings is showing solidarity with them, which is less common in societies characterized by greed, with extreme focus on individual success and economic achievements.

It is easier to make decisions about vaccines where the benefit to harm balance is less clear, like for the influenza and HPV vaccines, where my view is that mandatory vaccination cannot be justified, which I shall explain in the next chapters. The obligatory flu shot for children in New York illustrates that politicians can go too far. There is also a clear risk of corruption when something is mandated. A common argument for mandatory flu shots is that they prevent transmission of the virus to other people. However, there is no evidence that the vaccine does this, and when, in addition, it is unknown how many people die because of influenza (see next chapter), it will not even be possible to evaluate if taxpayers' money is well spent on coercive policies.[25]

We should avoid mandatory vaccination even if it is only indirect, like prohibiting access to school for unvaccinated children, which can stigmatize them and might handicap their possibilities in life, for example, if the parents resort to home schooling.

I admit that I am influenced by the many years I have researched psychiatric issues. I have come to the conclusion that forced admission and forced treatment do far more harm than good and should be prohibited by law, as the United Nations Convention on the Rights of Persons with Disabilities has called for.[26]

UNESCO's Universal Declaration on Bioethics and Human Rights states that "Any preventive, diagnostic and therapeutic medical intervention is only to be carried out with the prior, free and informed consent of the person concerned, based on adequate information. The consent should, where appropriate, be express and may be withdrawn by the person concerned at any time and for any reason without disadvantage or prejudice."[27] Accordingly, vaccines cannot be forced upon anybody, directly or indirectly, through deprivation of privileges the individual would otherwise have had (e.g., the right to go to school, to have a job, or to earn a living), all of which can be equated with coercion.

Actively refusing all vaccines is rare, around 1-2% in high-income countries.[28] It should therefore be possible to get close to 100% coverage for the most important vaccinations through dialogue and other interventions that do not involve punishment.

4

Influenza

Vaccination against influenza might seem obvious, but it isn't. It is controversial and illustrates that well-informed people may reach sound conclusions that go against official guidelines or mandates. I used influenza as one of the cases in my book *Survival in an Overmedicated World: Look Up the Evidence Yourself*, which is a self-help book aimed at teaching people how they can find reliable information on the Internet.[1] In this chapter, I have done the work for you.

When people say influenza, they mean influenza-like illness. Many virus infections can give influenza-like symptoms. The most relevant review of influenza vaccines is very large; it includes 52 clinical trials and over 80,000 people.[2] Inactivated vaccines reduced influenza in healthy adults from 2.3% to 0.9%, risk ratio 0.41 (0.36 to 0.47). This is a considerable effect at the population level, but the individual preventive effect is small: 71 healthy adults need to be vaccinated to prevent one of them from getting influenza. Furthermore, it is disappointing that vaccination did not decrease admissions to hospital, risk ratio 0.96 (0.85 to 1.08), or days off work (-0.04 days; -0.14 to 0.06).

There is a similar review of children.[3] Live attenuated influenza vaccines reduced influenza from 18% to 4%, risk ratio 0.22 (0.11 to 0.41). Only seven children would need to be vaccinated to prevent one case of influenza. The incidence of acute otitis media was similar following vaccine or placebo, risk ratio 0.98 (0.95 to 1.01). There was insufficient information to determine the effect on school absenteeism, whereas the vaccine might lead to fewer parents taking time off work, although the confidence interval included no effect, risk ratio 0.69 (0.46 to 1.03). Data on the most serious influenza complications leading to hospital admission were not available.

Inactivated vaccines reduced influenza in children from 30% to 11%, risk ratio 0.36 (0.28 to 0.48); only five children would need to be vaccinated to prevent one case of influenza. Again, the risk of otitis media was similar, 31% versus 27%; risk ratio 1.15 (0.95 to 1.40). There was insufficient information on school absenteeism and no data on parental working time lost or hospital admissions. One brand of monovalent pandemic vaccine caused sudden loss of muscle tone (cataplexy) and a sleep disorder (narcolepsy).[4]

It is widely believed among public health officials that vaccination saves many lives. But is it true or even likely, considering the lack of effect on hospital admission and lost workdays?

To address the possible effect on mortality, we could look for reviews of trials in frail people. In one such Cochrane review, there were eight trials in 5,000 people aged 65 and older.[5] Influenza over a single season was reduced from 6.0% to 2.4%, risk ratio 0.42 (0.27 to 0.66), but the strength of the evidence was low due to how influenza was diagnosed. These results indicated that 30 people would need to be vaccinated to prevent influenza in one person. Only one trial provided data for pneumonia and mortality. No cases of pneumonia occurred, and there were only three deaths among 522 participants in the vaccination arm and one among 177 participants in the placebo arm, risk ratio 1.02 (0.11 to 9.72). There were no data on hospital admissions.

In 2013, a group of researchers "rearranged" the data in the Cochrane review and found "substantial evidence for the ability of influenza vaccine to reduce the risk of influenza infection and influenza-related disease and death in the elderly."[6] A pretty amazing statistical stunt concluding that the vaccine reduces deaths when only four people died and the risk ratio was one! This paper was discussed at a Danish science site, and it was revealed that the corresponding author wrote the paper "after invitation from Cochrane."[7] This is problematic. The Cochrane Collaboration started as an idealistic grassroots organization, but it has developed in the wrong direction and is now too close to industry and other vested interests.[8] *BMJ*'s editor-in-chief, Fiona Godlee, wrote in 2018 that Cochrane should be committed to holding industry and academia to account, and that my expulsion from Cochrane reflects "a deep seated difference of opinion about how close to industry is too close."[9]

It was also revealed that the corresponding author on the Cochrane invited paper is notorious. Four years earlier, he had been accused of exaggerating the threat from swine flu because of his personal economic interests. His home country, Holland, bought a huge amount of vaccines in 2009, and it turned out that he owned 10% of the shares in the drug company ViroClinics B.V. This company announces on its website (in 2019):

"The clinical diagnostic testing services support and accelerate the market entry of new drugs, vaccines and antivirals, and assist in pre- and post-marketing surveillance programs. Services are customized to specific needs, enabling maximum flexibility from day-to-day analysis to high throughput bulk analysis."[10]

As I wanted to study the mortality, even though there were too few deaths in the trials to tell us anything, I googled *influenza vaccines lower mortality*. Already the top record was highly interesting.[11] The authors had tried to adjust for the inevitable bias caused by the fact that those who get vaccinated have another preexisting risk of dying compared with those who don't. They found that the mortality was low soon after vaccination and then increased over time in a pattern suggesting selection bias: "It is this rise in mortality with time since vaccination that is especially challenging in the estimation of vaccine effectiveness."

This study is far better than most other observational studies. The researchers included everyone aged 65 years or older who was a member of Kaiser Permanente in California and examined mortality before, during, and after nine flu seasons in relation to vaccination status from 1996 to 2005. The study was huge: a total of 115,823 deaths occurred, including 20,484 during laboratory-defined flu seasons, and vaccine coverage averaged 63%. It was therefore well suited to study mortality in relation to vaccination status.

The researchers' methods were very sophisticated, and they found a curvilinear relationship between predictors of mortality and vaccination status. Patients with heart disease, diabetes, or chronic obstructive pulmonary disease were more likely to get flu shots than other people. However, most such patients had only a moderately elevated risk of death, often in the range where vaccine coverage was highest. In higher-risk patients, vaccine coverage waned.

It seems plausible that near the end of life, frailty poses barriers to vaccination, and patients and doctors may give up on preventive measures. However, until then, patients with chronic conditions have more reason and opportunity to get vaccinated than healthy people, because such patients are more vulnerable to influenza and have more contacts with healthcare professionals who encourage vaccination.

Even though I admire this study, its level of sophistication made me anxious:

> We added polynomial terms for number of days since September 15, days squared, and days cubed in order to examine the trajectory of the odds ratio during the course of the flu year . . . Finally, we determined the average amount of excess (flu-attributable) mortality during flu season by fitting a Poisson regression model to data on 39,420 person-day strata (12 age-sex groups × 9 years × 365 calendar days, combining the 2 extra leap days with February 28). The count of deaths was regressed on a flu season indicator and covariates, with the person-time at risk included as an offset term. The covariates included number of days since September 15, days squared, an indicator for each flu year, and an indicator for each calendar month.[12]

Gosh! You might not have understood any of this, but you need not be familiar with statistics to realize that the more complicated a statistical model is, the less we know if the estimate of vaccine effectiveness is the most reliable one we could have obtained with the data. What I miss are the results of simpler models, which might have reassured me that the final estimate was reasonably reliable, if the various models did not yield results too far apart.

We may compare this with climate change. It has been studied in so many models, some much more sophisticated than others, and by so many different methods, with so many different data sets, that I don't have the slightest doubt that we humans are responsible for global warming and that it might end in disaster in the near future.

About their study's limitations, the researchers said that they might have missed flu shots given outside of Kaiser Permanente, e.g., delivered in nursing homes to patients near death. They also overlooked herd effects: non-vaccinated people might also benefit because their risk of getting infected is lowered. The researchers mentioned that they overlooked late effects "if the vaccine prevents complications that increase mortality after flu season." I would add that late effects can go both ways. As the commonly used influenza vaccine is not a live vaccine, it could increase total mortality (see Chapter 1).

The researchers noted as a limitation that their estimate depended on the severity of the flu seasons and the match of the vaccines to circulating strains of the virus. However, this is a limitation in all types of research, and also in randomized trials that have a nonvaccinated control group.

So, what was the effect of flu shots in the elderly? Virtually none. The researchers calculated that one death was prevented for every 4,000 people vaccinated. Furthermore, this estimate is very uncertain. The authors gave no confidence interval, but the lower end of this interval must be very close to no effect.

Such small effects in observational studies should not be believed. The biases, even after elaborate adjustments as in the current study, are often much larger than the estimated effect. Other studies have reported larger mortality reductions, but they are less reliable than the current study.[13]

We also need to consider the likelihood of getting infected without vaccination. Since pandemics are rare and rarely involve large portions of the population, the likelihood is very small. Further, as the virus mutates rapidly, we cannot be sure that the effect obtained by vaccination will be the same as in the randomized trials. We cannot even say what the risk of death is because some strains are more deadly than others.

Finally, we need to consider the harms of vaccination. If we use the estimate of one person avoiding death from influenza per 4,000 vaccinated, it means that 3,999 people will not benefit, and many of them will be harmed by the vaccination. Not serious harms, but the less the benefit, the more the harms count, both for the individual decision and when authorities issue recommendations.

Official Recommendations to Get Flu Shots Are Not Evidence-Based

I have never been vaccinated against influenza, and after having studied the evidence in detail, I am sure I never will. Several of my colleagues who are specialists in infectious diseases say the same, and so does my wife, who is a professor of Clinical Microbiology.

The advice from the authorities is totally different, and also bewildering. When I want to find out what the harms of drugs are, I often start by retrieving the package inserts from the Internet. Sometimes there is a long list of adverse events reported in the clinical trials on an active drug but no comparison with placebo. Caution is therefore needed when reading package inserts, as there can be a lot of noise. The best of them give you a good idea of which of the effects might be considered caused by the drug.

It is usually very easy to find the package inserts. For the depression pill duloxetine, googling *duloxetine fda* leads to the package insert as the top record, which has a black box warning in bold letters at the top of the first page:

> **WARNING: Suicidality and Antidepressant Drugs**
>
> *See full prescribing information for complete boxed warning.*
> - **Increased risk of suicidal thinking and behavior in children, adolescents, and young adults taking antidepressants for major depressive disorder (MDD) and other psychiatric disorders. Cymbalta is not approved for use in pediatric patients (5.1).**

I tried to do the same for influenza vaccines. I googled *influenza vaccine fda*, and while I was typing, Google suggested other options, of which the first was *influenza vaccine fda label.* The top record seemed to be a package insert, and the headline was *Influenza Virus Vaccine, Quadrivalent, Types A and Types B.*[14] However, I could not find any harms or warnings. The main entries were to the intranasal and the injectable vaccines, and to *Resources For You*, which had three subentries: *Influenza Virus Vaccine Safety*, *Licensed Biological Products with Supporting Documents*, and *Vaccines Licensed for Use in the United States.*

When I clicked on *Influenza Virus Vaccine Safety*, my surprise turned into suspicion. People wanting to find out what the adverse effects of influenza vaccines are would very likely find this link. Although the headline was *Influenza Virus Vaccine Safety & Availability*, it was not at all about informing people of the harms of the vaccines. It was pure propaganda of the kind usually only seen from drug companies. It went directly against what I have just documented above, and it shocked me so much that I will show you the full page:

> Influenza, also known as the flu, is a contagious respiratory disease that is caused by influenza viruses. Influenza viruses infect the respiratory tract (nose, throat, and lungs) in humans. The flu is different from a cold, mainly because the symptoms and complications are more severe. Influenza usually comes on suddenly and may include these symptoms: fever, headache, malaise (a feeling of being ill and without energy that can be extreme), cough, sore throat, nasal congestion and body aches.
>
> A lot of the illness and death caused by the influenza virus can be prevented by a yearly influenza vaccine. Most individuals 6 months of age and older should get the influenza vaccine every year. It is especially important for people in high-risk groups and people who are in close contact with those at

high risk to get an influenza vaccine every year as recommended by CDC's Advisory Committee on Immunization Practices (ACIP).

Influenza vaccine can be given to most individuals 6 months of age and older to protect against influenza. Persons who provide important community services (such as police, fire department personnel, emergency medical services) should consider getting an influenza vaccine so that those services are not disrupted during an influenza outbreak.

Seasonal Information
- Influenza Virus Vaccine Composition and Lot Release
- Importance of Influenza Vaccination for Health Care Personnel
- La Importancia de la Vacunación para el Personal Relacionado con el Cuidado de la Salud

Approved Vaccines
- Influenza Vaccine, Adjuvanted
- Influenza Virus Vaccine, Quadrivalent, Types A and Types B
- Influenza Virus Vaccine, Trivalent, Types A and B
- Influenza Virus Vaccine, H5N1 (for National Stockpile)

Related Information
- Pandemics & Emerging Diseases

Related Information from the Centers for Disease Control (CDC)
- Key Facts About Seasonal Flu Vaccine
- Preventing Seasonal Flu

Other Related Links
- www.Flu.gov
  One-stop access to US Government H1N1, avian, and pandemic flu information

It is unbelievable that the headline of this page was *Influenza Virus Vaccine Safety & Availability.* I was looking for safety, a euphemism for adverse effects or harms, but found nothing. FDA wrote that "A lot of the illness and death caused by the influenza virus can be prevented by a yearly influenza vaccine." This is simply not true, and the next sentence is: "Most individuals 6 months of age and older should get the influenza vaccine every year." The vaccine manufacturers couldn't have done such a marvelous job themselves. The FDA would have forbidden them to advertise that their vaccines reduce deaths, as this has not been documented (see FDA's sanctions against Roche's fanciful claims about Tamiflu in the next section).

Statements like "a lot of illness prevented" will be misinterpreted. Many people will think that their chance of benefiting from the vaccination exceeds 50%, but it is less than 2% because 71 healthy adults need to be vaccinated to prevent one of them from getting influenza.[15] Furthermore, the vaccine does not reduce admission to hospital or days off work, so what's the big deal?

That framing tactics, like the ones used by FDA, are highly misleading is illustrated by a study of thousands of women in nine European countries. They were asked in face-to-face interviews how many women out of 1,000 who participate every two years in mammography screening would have benefited after ten years, compared to women who did not participate in screening.[16] The response options were 0, 1, 10, 50, 100 and 200 per 1,000, and don't know. A fourth of all British women believed that 200 of every 1,000 women would be spared dying from breast cancer. The correct answer was 1 per 1,000, but the propaganda from the National Health Service has presented the benefit as a 20% reduction in mortality from breast cancer, which is likely the reason for the misperception. In the review of breast screening I have published and updated since 2001, we write that the trials were biased and explain that the three best trials did not find a statistically significant reduction in breast cancer mortality after 13 years, risk ratio 0.90 (0.79 to 1.02).[17]

Tamiflu and Relenza for Treating Influenza

Most people have heard about Tamiflu, the trade name for oseltamivir. We have wasted and still waste billions of any currency on this largely ineffective drug and a similar one, zanamivir (Relenza). A Cochrane review of the trials found that oseltamivir reduced the time to first alleviation of symptoms by 17 hours,[18] which is a small effect that might even be nonexistent. The trials were not effectively blinded because the drug has conspicuous side effects. The double-blind trials are therefore not truly double-blind because it is possible to guess correctly in many cases who gets active drug and who gets placebo. As it is highly subjective to say when influenza stops, the lack of blinding has likely rendered the result too positive.

More important, like for influenza vaccines, there were no certain effects on outcomes that matter—deaths, hospital admissions, pneumonia, any complication classified as serious, or reduced transmission of the virus to other people. The drug manufacturer Roche omitted publishing most of their clinical trial data and refused to share them with independent researchers.[19] Based on unpublished trials, Roche claimed that Tamiflu reduces hospital admissions by 61%, secondary complications by 67%, and lower respiratory tract infections requiring antibiotics by 55%. I consider that fraud.[20] Fraud means a wrongful or criminal deception intended to result in financial or personal gain, typically by unjustifiably claiming or being credited with accomplishments or qualities.

The FDA asked Roche to stop claiming that Tamiflu reduces the severity and incidence of secondary infections, while the European Medicines Agency accepted the claim that the drug reduces lower respiratory tract complications.

Zanamivir was rejected by FDA's advisory committee with the votes 13 to 4 because it was no better than placebo when patients were taking other drugs such as paracetamol. But after the company protested, FDA overruled its own committee and approved the drug, and therefore it also needed to approve oseltamivir later the same year.[21]

Many people wondered why WHO selected people to write guidance about influenza drugs who were paid by the companies selling the drugs and why this was not disclosed in their guidance reports. There was so much secrecy that it wasn't even possible for outsiders to get information about who was on the WHO committee.[22]

The scandals continued. In June 2009, WHO proclaimed the beginning of an influenza pandemic of the H1N1 swine flu virus, which soon proved to be an ordinary outbreak that was milder than those of the past. This was possible because a new definition of pandemics had been adopted just beforehand, despite protests by some of the Member States.[23] It has been estimated that 18 billion dollars were spent on the pandemic to vaccinate millions of people without it being clear whether the vaccine was useful, as it had never been tested clinically.[24]

During the ten years leading up to WHO's pandemic declaration of 2009, scientists associated with the companies that were to profit from WHO's "pandemic preparedness" programs, including Roche and GlaxoSmithKline, were involved at virtually every stage of the development of those programs.[25] Roy Anderson, a prominent British epidemiologist and adviser to both WHO and the UK government, gravely warned a BBC radio audience that only Relenza and Tamiflu would prevent a catastrophe on the scale of the 1918 influenza pandemic. At the time, Anderson was receiving £116,000 per year from GlaxoSmithKline, manufacturer of Relenza. By declaring a pandemic and linking the response to Tamiflu stockpiling, WHO could not have done a better job of promoting Roche's interests.

In 2008, an article in *Drug Safety* by a group of Roche authors claimed that rats and mice given a very high dose of Tamiflu showed no ill effect. But according to documents submitted to the Japanese Ministry of Health by Chugai, the Japanese Roche subsidiary, the exact same dose of Tamiflu killed more than half of the animals.[26] As they died, the rats exhibited many of the same central nervous system symptoms that a researcher had described in his case series on Japanese children. Moreover, cases of hallucination and weird accidents had been fairly commonly reported in Roche's postmarketing surveillance of Tamiflu.[27]

Following criticism of the CDC and its foundation for accepting a directed donation from Roche for the agency's Take 3 Flu Campaign, which encouraged the public to "take antiviral medicine if your doctor prescribes it," the CDC posted an article on its website titled "Why CDC recommends influenza antiviral drugs."[28] The agency cited multiple observational and industry-funded studies, including a meta-analysis described as "independent," even though it was sponsored by Roche. All four authors had financial ties to Roche, Genentech, or Gilead. Despite its extensive list of studies, the CDC article did not cite the Cochrane review even though it had also been published in the *BMJ*, one of the best and most well-known medical journals in the world.[29]

The CDC director told the public that these drugs could "save your life," which looked like classic stealth marketing where the industry places messages in the mouths of trusted third parties. There is no reliable evidence that these drugs save lives, and it is highly unlikely that they do.

Oseltamivir causes psychiatric adverse events, headaches, renal events, nausea, and vomiting. I would not take this drug or zanamivir should I get influenza.

Any Reason to Vaccinate Healthcare Workers?

The FDA page about safety did not tell us anything about safety but recommended service people get vaccinated.[30] Does this reduce the risk of transmission of the virus to other people? As there was no information about this in the large Cochrane review,[31] I googled *does influenza vaccine prevent transmission?* The top record was an article on the CDC website, "Vaccine effectiveness: how well do the flu vaccines work?"[32] I found nothing there about preventing transmission, only high praises of the vaccine, so I continued searching. Farther down on the Google page, there was information for healthcare workers from the CDC: "The findings of a CDC review of related published literature indicate that influenza vaccination of health care personnel can enhance patient safety." [33] There were two references; one to a systematic CDC review from 2014, the other to an editorial commenting on that review.[34]

Already the introduction to the review makes it clear that it is controversial whether vaccination of healthcare personnel reduces morbidity and mortality among patients. Two recent systematic reviews were cited: one concluded that there is likely a protective effect for patients in long-term care settings; the other that there is a lack of evidence. The CDC review (four of its five authors worked at the CDC) included four cluster randomized trials, two cohort studies, and two case-control studies. That made me somewhat skeptical. Drug regulators require randomized trials for drug approval, as this is the only research design that can tell us reliably what drugs do to people, and these trials are usually placebo-controlled to make the outcome assessment more reliable.

The burden of proof for efficacy must be particularly high in a situation where people—the healthcare workers—do not take a drug to benefit themselves, but to benefit others. Cohort studies, where groups who have or haven't taken a drug are being compared, are too unreliable to tell us anything about efficacy unless the effect is very large. There are many reasons why two groups assembled without randomization are not comparable and people who get vaccinated do not have the same health status as those who don't.[35] Case-control studies, where for example dead and living people are being compared as to whether they have been vaccinated, are even more unreliable.

The four cluster randomized trials presented data on 116 long-term care facilities randomized to vaccination and control arms. Thus, all healthcare workers in the same facility were either vaccinated or not vaccinated. This arrangement created very small sample sizes, only 15 institutions per trial in each arm, on average. With such small sample sizes, randomization cannot ensure that the compared groups were comparable to begin with. The authors acknowledged this problem and that they could not rule out bias due to different patterns of circulation of viruses within intervention and control facilities.

The mean age of the patients ranged from 77 to 86 years. Reported healthcare personnel vaccination rates ranged from 48% to 70% in the intervention arms and from 5% to 32% in the control arms. Thus, it seemed that some staff had already been vaccinated before the trial started, or the trial protocol had been violated in many cases because staff members who were not supposed to get vaccinated got vaccinated while the trial was running.

The results are unconvincing. The risk ratio for all-cause mortality was 0.71 (0.59 to 0.85), indicating a 29% (15% to 41%) reduction in deaths. However, the authors questioned this result because influenza has been estimated to contribute to less than 10% of all winter deaths among persons aged 65 years and older. Thus, even if the vaccine had been 100% effective in preventing influenza deaths, the reduction in total deaths should have been less than 10%. Furthermore, the vaccine almost always consists of inactivated virus, and Aaby's studies suggest this increases all-cause mortality (see Chapter 1). The result is therefore highly implausible.

For influenza-like illness, the risk ratio was 0.58 (0.46 to 0.73), whereas there were no statistically significant effects on hospital admission, risk ratio 0.91 (0.61 to 1.19), or on laboratory-confirmed influenza, risk ratio 0.80 (0.31 to 2.08).

One should not require healthcare workers to get vaccinated without knowing whether this leads to fewer hospital admissions or complications to influenza, and the result for total mortality should be ignored.

It is inexcusable that the CDC on its website does not mention the relevant Cochrane review about influenza vaccination for healthcare workers who care for the elderly in long-term care institutions, first published in 2006 and updated in 2010, 2013, and 2016.[36] The 2016 version is 60 sixty pages and is so detailed that it allows readers to judge whether they agree with the authors. CDC searched for studies in the Cochrane Library, quoted Cochrane tools and the Cochrane Handbook for Systematic Reviews, and used Cochrane software for their meta-analyses. It therefore seems deliberate that they ignored the Cochrane review and preferred to quote their own review, although it is far less rigorous than the Cochrane review.

I have come across this practice many times. National boards of health, drug agencies, and other authorities prefer to quote substandard research and to ignore better research that questions the basis for their political agenda or disagrees with what their funders—the politicians who have the power to strip the funding—expect of them. My worst experience is related to mammography screening. The Danish Board of Health consistently referred to very poor research whose results were politically expedient rather than to our far more rigorous research, which was published in top journals. I have done a lot of research in this area, and the distortion of the truth, also by pro-mammography researchers, which even involved fraud, was so pervasive that I wrote a whole book about it with a title similar to this book's.[37]

The Cochrane review states in the abstract that influenza vaccination is not very effective: "A systematic review found that 3% of working adults who had received influenza vaccine and 5% of those who were unvaccinated had laboratory-proven influenza per season."[38]

It included the same four trials as those in the CDC review. The principal sources of bias in the trials were related to attrition, lack of blinding, vaccination in the control groups, and low rates of vaccination coverage in the intervention arms, which led the authors to downgrade the quality of evidence for all outcomes due to serious risk of bias. They did not find any information on cointerventions with healthcare worker vaccination: hand-washing, face masks, early detection of laboratory-proven influenza, quarantine, avoiding admissions, antivirals, and asking healthcare workers with influenza or influenza-like illness not to work. All such measures might have biased the trials toward finding an effect of vaccination. None of the trials explicitly stated that they had appropriate means of blinding participants or study personnel to vaccination, but two trials mentioned that the study nurses were informed if any patient developed symptoms of influenza or took additional opportunistic nose and throat swabs from such patients. This might have increased the incidence of laboratory-proven influenza in the nonvaccinated group.

There was no statistically significant effect of vaccination on laboratory-proven influenza, risk difference 0 (-0.03 to 0.03), lower respiratory tract infection, risk difference -0.02 (-0.04 to 0.01; it went down from 6% to 4% in one study of 3400 people), or admission to hospital for respiratory illness, risk difference 0 (-0.02 to 0.02). The authors decided not to combine data on deaths from lower respiratory tract infection or from all causes because the direction and size of difference in risk varied between the studies. They were also uncertain as to the effect of vaccination on these outcomes due to the very low quality of evidence. They concluded that their review did not provide reasonable evidence to support the vaccination of healthcare workers to prevent influenza in elderly care-demanding people.

I agree. There are far too many uncertainties in the four trials. The editorial accompanying the CDC review was also critical and highlighted additional findings that did not make sense.[39] The authors estimated a 42% reduction in influenza-like illness, whereas the reduction in the more specific outcome, laboratory-confirmed influenza, wasn't higher than this but only 20%. Another concern was that the risk reduction in death was greater (40%) when the analysis included a broader time period than when the analysis was confined to the period when influenza was circulating (22%). If the homes were appropriately balanced through the randomization process, and vaccination provided protection, one would expect to find the greatest effects during influenza periods.

Canadian researchers recently reviewed the evidence and agreed with the Cochrane researchers.[40] There is no valid evidence to support the hypothesis that vaccinating healthcare workers protects patients from influenza. One researcher mentioned that vaccination for the H3N2 subtype resulted in a vaccine effectiveness of around 40%, which means that three out of five vaccinated healthcare workers remain as susceptible to H3N2 as if they were unvaccinated. She added: "In that context, to focus exclusively on the risk posed by unvaccinated workers—treating them as outcasts or, worse, terminating their employment—while overlooking the risk posed by vaccinated workers, potentially jeopardizes patients."[41]

Indeed. Vaccination may provide staff with a false sense of security, which might reduce their level of handwashing and potentially increase, rather than decrease, the risk of infecting patients. We need a large, high-quality trial if we wish to know whether vaccination of healthcare workers benefits those they care for. Yet it is unlikely that it will show tangible benefits, and, as I have argued in the previous chapter, it is unethical to request healthcare workers to run a personal risk of getting seriously harmed in order to possibly protect others. I would therefore find such a trial unethical.

The CDC recommends that all US healthcare workers get vaccinated annually against influenza.[42] Of course they do. They might lose funding if they didn't.

Other Misleading CDC Messages

Many messages on official websites are seriously misleading. It is an unfathomable pollution of our common scientific knowledge to propagate all this misinformation and clear it with a seemingly respectable governmental rubber stamp. I shall give some further examples.

The CDC website is a treasure trove of misinformation, even worse than what I have seen on drug company websites. It announces colossal effects of vaccination without the slightest hint that these estimates come from highly unreliable research such as case-control studies. In responsible medical research, this would not be accepted, e.g., breast-screening experts have agreed that case-control studies cannot say anything reliably about the effect of screening.[43] The bias can be huge, as demonstrated by data from the Malmö randomized breast-screening trial. When properly analyzed as a randomized trial, there was no reduction in breast-cancer mortality, risk ratio 0.96 (0.68 to 1.35). When analyzed as a case-control study, comparing breast-cancer mortality in attenders with nonattenders within the screening arm, the odds ratio was 0.42 (0.22 to 0.78).[44] Thus a nonsignificant reduction in breast-cancer mortality of 4% became a significant but false reduction of 58%. The flaw is called the "healthy screenee effect," i.e., those who attend screening have less risk of dying from breast cancer than those who don't. Some women may avoid screening because they fear something may be wrong with them, and women from lower socioeconomic groups also often choose not to be screened and have higher mortality from a range of diseases, including breast cancer.

The CDC website about vaccine effectiveness illustrates the pervasiveness of the misinformation.[45] The link for this interesting information, "During 2016–2017, flu vaccination prevented an estimated 85,000 flu-related hospitalizations," did not work. I landed on a page with this text: "Oops! We can't seem to find the page you were looking for. Please try our search or A–Z index." I searched and searched, but even just a search on *85,000* led nowhere, as the search button was dead. I then used the A–Z index and went to *Influenza Vaccination*. On that page, I could see at the top that in the most recent flu season, 2018–2019, there had been about 40 million flu illnesses, 600,000 flu hospitalizations and 36,400–61,200 flu deaths. Wow! Seven times as many hospitalizations as in 2016–2017; perhaps this was why the more modest number was removed. Large numbers of casualties are used in scare campaigns. If we, for example, want to find out whether depression pills work and look up an official website that, as its first information, says that over 10% of the US population currently suffers from depression (which is correct, given the far too loose criteria for what it takes to get a depression diagnosis),[46] then we have no doubt that the underlying message is that we should use depression pills to combat the "disaster."

I refused to give up and searched for *85,000* on the *Influenza Vaccination* page: 330 search results. *Flu-related hospitalizations* returned 1,334 results, or 460 when I used quotation marks. Then I tried *prevented an estimated 85,000 flu-related hospitalizations*, which yielded 7 results. Some of these were identical, but there were 4 unique links: *Key Facts About Seasonal Flu Vaccine | CDC*; *Misconceptions about Seasonal Flu and Flu Vaccines | CDC*; *What are the benefits of flu vaccination?* | *CDC*; and *Vaccine Effectiveness: How Well Do the Flu Vaccines Work?* | *CDC*. When I opened each of these links and searched on *85,000*, I ended up each time on the *Oops!* page.

It was like getting lost in a forest. After many hours of walking, you realize you went around in a circle and are back to where you started. I gave up on this hide-and-seek exercise that banged me back to square one every time and went to my next ordeal: "A 2014 study [external icon] showed that flu vaccine reduced children's risk of flu-related pediatric intensive care unit (PICU) admission by 74% during flu seasons from 2010-2012."[47] What an impressive result! And no playing games this time; the link was to a published study.[48] Considering the findings in the randomized trials, the result was totally implausible, but this trifle had not led the authors to provide any reservations in their abstract. It was a case-control study where the cases were admitted to an intensive care unit with severe respiratory illness and testing positive for influenza. The controls were children in an intensive care unit who tested negative, and there were also community controls. These groups were compared for vaccination status.

"Vaccine effectiveness was estimated with logistic regression models." This woke me up. I have some knowledge of statistics, and I plowed through heavy textbooks of statistics when I did my doctoral thesis and made three-way analyses of variance on a pocket calculator because I had not yet bought my first computer. The study continued:

> The regression model used to compare cases to PICU controls included the natural log of age in months, gender, time of illness onset (pre-, peak, or post-peak influenza period), reported contact with a person with suspected or confirmed influenza, history of moderate to severe respiratory disorders (excluding mild asthma), history of cardiac disorders, illness severity on admission (PRISM Score [37]), days between illness onset and influenza testing, and a dichotomous variable indicating if enrolment occurred outside active recruitment. We adjusted for geographic area by including site as a random effect.[49]

It is not helpful to do so many adjustments in a model because it has been documented that the more variables you include in a logistic regression, the further you are likely to get from the truth.[50] This study should be forgotten and should never have made it to an official website.

The CDC provided more entertainment: "In recent years, flu vaccines have reduced the risk of flu-associated hospitalizations among adults on average by about 40%."[51] How is this possible when the randomized trials didn't find anything? Oh well, it was a systematic review of case-control studies. Forget it.

"A 2018 study showed that from 2012 to 2015, flu vaccination among adults reduced the risk of being admitted to an intensive care unit (ICU) with flu by 82 percent."[52] Interesting game. We are approaching 100% vaccine efficacy but are witnessing a scientific playroom, totally detached from reality. The study used methods similar to the one on children discussed just above,[53] and there was an element of recycling, as Thompson from CDC (not the so-called whistleblower Thompson from Chapter 2) coauthored three of the studies.[54]

CDC's hoopla just continued: "Flu vaccine can be life-saving in children. A 2017 study was the first of its kind to show that flu vaccination can significantly reduce a child's risk of dying from influenza."[55] The link was to a CDC press release that didn't reveal the source. Hide-and-seek again. But this time it was easy to find it, in a Google search (I didn't dare do any more searches on the CDC website), as the press release started with "A new CDC study published today in *Pediatrics*. . ."[56] The authors had conducted a case-cohort analysis using logistic regression. Vaccine effectiveness was estimated to be 65%. Again, highly implausible, and again using methods similar to those in the other highly unreliable studies.

We were also told that vaccination has led to lower rates of some cardiac events among people with heart disease and to reduced hospitalizations among people with diabetes and chronic lung disease. Of course. Deeply flawed research can give us any result we want.

So, what did the CDC say about the flaws in the unreliable studies it presented on its website? Absolutely nothing.[57] It explained that:

> Randomized studies are the "gold standard" (best method) for determining how well a vaccine works. The effects of vaccination measured in these studies is called "efficacy." Randomized, placebo controlled studies are expensive and are not conducted after a recommendation for vaccination has been issued, as withholding vaccine from people recommended for vaccination would place them at risk for infection, illness and possibly serious complications. For that reason, most U.S. studies conducted to determine the benefits of flu vaccination are "observational studies." "Observational studies" compare the occurrence of flu illness in vaccinated people compared to unvaccinated people, based on their decision to be vaccinated or not. This means that vaccination of study subjects is not randomized. The measurement of vaccine effects in an observational study is referred to as "effectiveness."[58]

It is astonishing that the CDC can write so much about the two types of study design playing with the words *efficacy* and *effectiveness*, as if this would make any difference, without saying anything about the fact that observational studies are generally unreliable when estimating benefits.

More Impressive but Misleading Numbers

Here is another example of how seriously it can go wrong in case-control studies. Spanish researchers reported in their abstract that, compared with patients who were unvaccinated in the current and three previous seasons, influenza vaccination in the current and any previous season reduced mortality by 70% (34% to 87%).[59] They also wrote that "Vaccination in the current season only had no significant effect on cases of severe influenza." This would lead readers to conclude that people should be vaccinated every year in order to become adequately protected, and this was also how the researchers interpreted their data: "These results reinforce recommendations for annual vaccination for influenza in older adults." However, the main text of the paper noted that, "vaccination in the current season only showed no reduced odds of severe disease and increased odds of death" (adjusted odds ratio of 3.35 [1.06 to 10.58]). They wrote that this was consistent with a preventive effect against nonsevere influenza, but not against severe influenza.

This explanation does not make sense. The authors touted a huge effect of the vaccine on mortality, 70% (which is totally implausible), and then say that the vaccine does not work against severe influenza. It is severe influenza, not mild disease, that kills people.

*   *   *

It has never been shown in reliable research that flu shots reduce deaths. But we are bombarded with highly misleading information, not only about the effect, but also about the number of influenza deaths, the purpose of which is to scare people into getting vaccinated.

The Canadian Broadcasting Corporation (CBC) reported that, in 2012, the Public Health Agency of Canada said in a press release: "Every year, between 2,000 and 8,000 Canadians die of the flu and its complications."[60] The editor of the *Canadian Medical Association Journal* joined the requiem and repeated the "up to 8,000 people" statement.

No one knows how many people die after being infected with the flu virus. The numbers are not based on body counts, lab tests, or autopsies; they are based on computer models.[61]

One model counts all respiratory and circulatory deaths, including people who died of a heart attack that had nothing to do with flu. Another model assumes that every extra death that happens in the winter is a flu death. Thus, the basic idea is that winter deaths—even deaths from slippery sidewalks, snowy roads, and freezing temperatures—minus summer deaths equals flu deaths. Flu deaths even include deaths from psychotic conditions.

Models are highly sensitive to the assumptions you feed into them. And what about a person who is already extremely fragile with heart or lung disease and who is tipped over the edge with a flu infection: is that a flu death, a heart death, or a lung death? Impossible to say.

In contrast to the claimed 8,000 deaths, there were only about 300 deaths a year in Statistics Canada's mortality table under *cause of death: influenza*.

A researcher used data from three Ottawa hospitals over seven flu seasons and counted the patients who died from flu, according to a doctor's diagnosis. When she ran one of the official computer models, it predicted eight times as many deaths from flu as there were actual clinical cases!

When the CBC journalist contacted the researcher, he was told that he needed to contact the Public Health Agency of Canada even if he was just looking for background information, as she worked for the Agency.

His request for permission to talk to the researcher about her master's thesis was directed all the way up to the chief of media relations for Health Canada. The journalist noted in an email that he needed some background for a story he was doing; that the researcher was interested in talking to him; and that he would not be speaking to her as a representative of a government agency, but only as the author of a student thesis.

The chief of media relations wrote back that he had spoken with the student who "would prefer that you quote from her written thesis as her current workload doesn't leave her a lot of extra time these days." He offered the journalist a chance to ask about the official government point of view and suggested that a media relations officer contact him. An on-camera interview with anyone from Health Canada about any of this was refused, however.

When the so-called flu pandemic hit in 2009, and WHO had scared the whole world about how serious this would likely be, a rare opportunity arose to check the true death toll from flu. For the first time, there was widespread lab testing, a national reporting system, and all eyes were on potential flu-related deaths. The final count, 428 deaths, was much closer to the seasonal average of around 300 recorded in the vital statistics tables than to the up-to-8,000 deaths estimated with the computer models.[62]

Instead of scaring us, health officials could assure us that we shouldn't be worried. Even the wildly exaggerated estimate of 8,000 could be turned around to almost nothing. It means that 99.98% of Canadians would *not* die of flu during a year. The 428 deaths correspond to only 0.15% of all annual deaths in Canada. In contrast, 17% die of tobacco smoking, which is over 100 times as many. If we want to lower the number of deaths, we should focus on stopping smoking and preventing young people from ever starting. In Norway, high taxes have had a dramatic effect. Cigarettes are twice the cost of those in Denmark, and only 3% of young people smoke, compared to 15% in Denmark.[63] Why, then, all this propaganda about flu shots? We don't even know whether flu shots decrease deaths.

The Canadian models have pushed the estimated number of deaths upward all the time. Around the year 2000, the upper end of the estimate was 1,500, which increased to 2,500 in 2003, and to 8,000 in 2007. Flu researcher Tom Jefferson, whose Cochrane reviews I cite in this book, said: "Influenza prevention has become an industry fueled by poor science and propelled by conflicted decision makers. . . . How many die every year? Answer: maybe 300 or maybe 9,000. We are not sure. If you do not know, how can you have such a costly policy and most of all how can you evaluate it? . . . Scaring people justifies evidence-free policies. . . . The only certainty are the returns for industry."

The CBC journalist had asked the Public Health Agency why it was important to inform Canadians about the death statistics. The official, written response was:

> Reporting on these death statistics informs Canadians that infection with influenza can be severe and in some cases result in death. Hence, Canadians should get their seasonal flu shot to prevent infection and to practice infection control measures such as hand washing, cough etiquette and staying home when sick to prevent spread.[64]

Why is it that public health officials so often seriously manipulate the evidence in order to scare people to do what they recommend? There should be stiff penalties for such scientific misconduct. Do they get a bonus depending on the number of flu shots per year? Sometimes people do, e.g., Danish police chiefs are being rewarded after the number of traffic fines their subordinates deliver. In healthcare, the bonus is likely indirect. By howling with the wolves and pleasing the politicians, you can look forward to a rewarding career in public health.

The logic in public health is that if many people die from a disease (even though we don't know this but just assume it), we should try to prevent some of the deaths (even though we have no intervention with a documented effect). I shall give another example of this faulty reasoning.

We demonstrated in 2012 that general health checks, called annual physicals in the United States, don't work. We updated our review in 2019 and added one more trial.[65] The median follow-up was long, ten years, and there were 21,535 deaths in the randomized trials, which is a lot. Health checks did not lower total mortality, risk ratio 1.00 (0.97 to 1.03), cardiovascular mortality, risk ratio 1.01 (0.92 to 1.12), or cancer mortality, risk ratio 1.05 (0.94 to 1.16).

The United Kingdom had health checks already in 2012 with screening for several diseases. The official replies to our review were so bizarre that I called them a soap opera.[66] I wrote an article in the *BMJ* titled "I don't want the truth, I want something I can tell Parliament!":

> Public Health England will establish an expert panel to review the effectiveness and value for money of NHS Health Checks, and it will refresh the economic modelling behind the programme. We are furthermore told that 'although we recognise that the programme is not supported by direct randomised controlled trial evidence, there is nonetheless an urgent need to tackle the growing burden of disease which is associated with lifestyle behaviours and choices.'[67]

The truth, that health checks don't work and are likely harmful, is too much to bear for Public Health England, it seems. An expert panel is the modern version of the Oracle in Delphi, and statistical modeling is like whispering in a wizard's ear which result you would like to hear. Saying that there is an urgent need to tackle the growing burden of disease as an excuse for going against clear evidence from randomized trials reminds me of another episode of "Yes, Minister" where it was skillfully argued why a huge number of administrators were needed for a hospital that had no patients.[68]

So, the burden of a disease is what sets public health in motion. Whether what is done works or not doesn't matter. Political expediency is about doing *something*, not about doing *nothing*.

Vaccination during Pregnancy

What does the CDC say about pregnancy? "Vaccination reduces the risk of flu-associated acute respiratory infection in pregnant women by up to one-half" and "A 2018 study showed that getting a flu shot reduced a pregnant woman's risk of being hospitalized with flu by an average of 40 percent."[69] Case-control studies again, by the same nonwhistleblower Thompson from the CDC I have already mentioned.[70] Forget about them.

The CDC page said: "Getting vaccinated can also protect a baby after birth from flu. (Mom passes antibodies onto the developing baby during her pregnancy.) A number of studies have shown that in addition to helping to protect pregnant women, a flu vaccine given during pregnancy helps protect the baby from flu infection for several months after birth, when he or she is not old enough to be vaccinated."

The link was to a page called *Pregnant Women & Influenza (Flu)* where there were references to seven studies. One was a report of two random-ized placebo-controlled trials in South Africa that included 2116 pregnant women who were not infected with HIV and 194 who were infected.[71] For the pregnant women who received placebo, and also for their babies, the infection rate for laboratory confirmed influenza was 3.6%, while 1.8% and 1.9%, respectively, were infected when the woman was vaccinated with inactivated influenza vaccine, i.e., the effect of the vaccine was about 50%. The vaccination was effective up until 24 weeks after birth. Two versus zero mothers died.

This study confirms that the vaccine is not particularly effective and there are some interesting data in an 88-page supplement to the paper that few people will ever read, which have been analyzed in a systematic review.[72] The study did not find significant differences between the two groups in maternal hospitalization for any infection, risk ratio 2.27 (0.94 to 5.49), or for neonatal hospitalization for sepsis, risk ratio 1.60 (0.73 to 3.50). However, while the differences were not statistically significant, the results were in favor of no vaccination. The results for infant deaths went in the opposite direction: 15 vs. 21 deaths.

The supplement furthermore shows that there were about 26 times as many cases of influenza-like illness as of influenza in the infants, and the vaccine had no effect on these (efficacy rate of 0.6%). It can be argued that a reduction in influenza is of limited value, if the net burden of influenza-like illness (including influenza) is not decreased.[73]

Is it safe to vaccinate pregnant women? There were 1062 non-HIV-infected women in the vaccine group and 1054 in the placebo group.

Miscarriage (before 28 weeks): 3 vs. 5, stillbirth (at 28 weeks or later): 15 vs. 9, preterm birth (before 37 weeks): 108 vs. 96. I calculated that these minor differences are not statistically significant, which is reassuring (p is 0.30 for stillbirth and 0.56 for premature birth). As the placebo group received saline, and not an immunogenic adjuvant, which is usually the case in vaccine trials, we can trust that the minor increase in adverse events in the vaccine group was not underestimated.

The CDC webpage mentioned two other randomized trials, one of which was large.[74] In Nepal, 3,693 pregnant women were allocated to inactivated vaccine or a saline placebo. The protective effect of the vaccine was 19% for influenza-like illness in the mothers and 30% for laboratory-confirmed influenza in the infants. There were fewer babies with low birth weight (less than 2,500 g) in the vaccination group, 23% vs. 27% (p = 0.02). Miscarriage occurred in 5 vs. 3 cases, stillbirth in 33 vs. 31, and congenital defects in 1.1% vs. 1.0%. Three vs. five women and 61 vs. 50 infants age 0–6 months died. No serious adverse events were associated with receipt of immunization.

The CDC webpage ends with this recommendation, in bold:

> **Getting vaccinated yourself may also protect people around you, including those who are more vulnerable to serious flu illness, like babies and young children, older people, and people with certain chronic health conditions.[75]**

It has not been documented that vaccination of pregnant women protects others against serious infection. But even for pregnant women, the evidence is less clear than we would have wanted. The CDC did not mention a large trial in 4,193 third-trimester pregnant women in Mali,[76] which compared trivalent inactivated influenza vaccine with quadrivalent meningococcal vaccine, which is also a nonlive vaccine. It is not ideal to have an active control group, but it is of interest that serious presumed neonatal infection was more common in infants in the influenza vaccine group than in the meningococcal vaccine group (60 vs. 37; p = 0.02) and that there was a tendency toward more infant deaths (52 vs. 37, p = 0.13).

If we add up the infant deaths in the two large placebo-controlled trials, we get 76 in the vaccine groups and 71 in the placebo groups, which is reassuring. If we add the deaths from the trial in Mali, we get 128 vs. 108, which is less reassuring. The meningococcal vaccine might have reduced deaths, but according to the first author, no one died from meningitis, and since it is not a live vaccine, it would not be expected to reduce deaths via nonspecific effects.

What Are the Harms of Flu Shots?

As noted above, the first two CDC websites I found did not say anything useful about the harms of flu shots.[77] One would expect *Influenza vaccination information for health care workers*[78] to say something meaningful about the harms, but it didn't. It devoted only 45 of its 3,622 words to this:

> **Flu vaccines are safe.** Serious problems from a flu vaccine are very rare. The most common side effect that a person is likely to experience is soreness where the injection was given. This is generally mild and usually goes away after a day or two.

This message ended with: "Visit Influenza Vaccine Safety for more information." I clicked on the link and got this message: "Unable to open [website address]. Cannot locate the Internet server or proxy server."

By now, I had lost my patience with the CDC. It felt like the CDC had ensured that no one would ever find anything about the harms of flu shots. It might just have been a technical problem that occurs when people rearrange websites and forget to correct the links. But the unspoken message I got out of all my troubles, and after having seen so much untrustworthy propaganda, was: "Don't ask questions, just do as we tell you and vaccinate all your patients every year, from 6 months to the grave. We already told you that flu vaccines are safe, so what's your problem?"

Mild soreness at the injection site for a day or two? Is this really everything there is to say about the harms of a flu shot?

The first FDA website I found was even worse than the CDC's because *Influenza Virus Vaccine Safety & Availability* had no information about safety.[79] Why did these agencies conceal the harms? Facing dead ends at two major US agencies raises concerns. Other agencies and institutions, be it drug agencies, ministries of health, boards of health, or WHO, aren't interested either in telling people honestly what we know about the harms of vaccines and what we don't know but would like to know. And questions are unwelcome. I regard this as unsolicited paternalism. I never gave my permission to let others decide for me whether I should get vaccinated, and with which vaccines, or to hide uncomfortable information.

Having come so far in my explorations made me angry. I now understood very clearly why some people are skeptical toward vaccines and may become irrational. Who can they believe? And are they covering up something? Public health has gone way too far with its "Daddy knows best" attitude, and the arrogance has backfired.

After all my involuntary detours, I tried one last one. I explained earlier that when I clicked on *Influenza Virus Vaccine Safety* on the CDC website, I found nothing about safety, only untrustworthy propaganda for the vaccine. I got a weird idea. I googled *Influenza Virus Vaccine Safety CDC*. I expected to get nowhere, but there was something about safety, both for patients and professionals,[80] two more clicks away. Four different types of vaccines were listed: inactivated influenza vaccine, cell culture-based inactivated influenza vaccine, recombinant influenza vaccine, and live, attenuated influenza vaccine. I looked up the inactivated one. Under adverse events were listed: "Pain and other injection site reactions: Up to 65% of people vaccinated experience pain at the injection site during the first week after vaccination which usually did not interfere with activity." Aha. This is far worse than the mild soreness for a day or two, which the CDC informed about on a website one can easily find. Not much consistency there. And other injection site reactions are not just pain, which the trial from South Africa illustrated. It reported that injection site reactions (mainly mild to moderate) were more frequent with the vaccine than with the placebo vaccine and that there were no other significant differences between the two study groups.[81] However, the supplementary appendix gave another impression. I found three major flaws in the tables, which all tended to underestimate the harms. First, data were given for non-HIV infected and HIV-infected women separately, which makes no sense, as local reactions are independent of HIV status; the two groups should therefore have been combined. Second, although the reactions were divided into mild, moderate, and severe, the tests used for deciding whether there were statistically significant differences between the vaccine and the placebo were applied on each severity category separately. A correct test would have been, for example, a chi-square test for trend (when there are three ordered groups, one must, of course, do a trend test and not overlook the ordering). Third, there were only data from 536 of the 2,310 randomized women (23%). I could not find any explanation why data from 77% of the women were missing. Since the article spoke about "The details of solicited local and systemic reactions," it seems that all women were asked about harms, so why were there only data for 23% of them?

These flaws reduce substantially the trial's ability to detect differences between the vaccine and the placebo in local and systematic harms. Since the trial was published in a highly prestigious journal, *New England Journal of Medicine*, it may seem surprising that the editors let the authors get away with this, but it is not surprising.

I looked up whether the authors had conflicts of interest, and they did. Their study was supported by the Bill and Melinda Gates Foundation (see Chapter 1), the vaccine was purchased from Sanofi Pasteur, and the first author had numerous conflicts of interest in relation to vaccine manufacturers including Sanofi Pasteur.

New England Journal of Medicine is also conflicted. It earns huge amounts of money from selling reprints of trial reports and advertisements to drug companies. So much so that it would not tell us anything about it when we asked and even refused to tell us which percentage of its income comes from reprints.[82]

I have described the editors' role in the Vioxx scandal elsewhere.[83] Merck cheated with the data on heart attacks caused by Vioxx, an arthritis drug, in a pivotal trial. The editors blamed Merck and the clinical investigators but forgot to mention their own role in allowing the obviously flawed paper to appear in print. After five years of silence, when the drug had been withdrawn and the journal ran the risk of getting accused in court cases, the editors finally reacted by publishing what they euphemistically called an "expression of concern." If they had acted earlier, it might have killed the sales of Vioxx instead of killing the patients, as the journal is so influential, and it would also have blunted the impact of reprint sales. *New England Journal of Medicine* sold 929,400 reprints of the article—more than one for every doctor in the Unites States —and they brought in between $697,000 and $836,000. The journal's owner, Massachusetts Medical Society, listed $88 million in total publishing revenue for just one year. Most of this likely comes from *New England Journal of Medicine*. I have estimated that Vioxx has killed about 120,000 people, most of whom didn't even need the drug but could have fared well with a nonlethal pain killer or without any drug at all.[84]

In the South African flu vaccine trial,[85] there were also more cases in the vaccine groups than in the placebo groups of erythema, swelling, induration, bruising, itching, joint pain, and muscle pain. These harms are signals that need to be taken seriously. I have spoken to colleagues who—encouraged by their hospitals to take the vaccines to protect the patients—developed severe itching, swelling, and induration, which was totally unexpected for them because they thought the vaccine was harmless. This doesn't happen if you just have a blood sample taken.

A placebo control with saline was not needed in the trial. When you ask patients whether they have experienced local reactions after a saline injection, some will affirm this, but you won't ask if they did not receive an injection. As an example of what this means, 49 of 181 non-HIV-infected women reported induration at the injection site in the vaccine group and 22 of 172 in the placebo group. If placebo had not been used, these numbers should have been 49 versus zero.

The CDC website noted other harms:

> Fever, malaise, myalgia, and other systemic symptoms can occur, most often affecting individuals who have had no previous exposure to the influenza virus antigens in the vaccine (e.g., young children). In adults, the rate of having these symptoms is similar after the vaccine and after a placebo injection.[86]

I am convinced that placebo *does not* give the same symptoms as the vaccine. Some people I have spoken to fell ill after a flu shot with inactivated vaccine and had pretty bad experiences. It is possible, of course, that they merely contracted a virus infection at the same time. But what does "similar" rate mean after a placebo injection? Was the rate higher in the vaccine group but numbers too low to make the difference statistically significant like in the South African trial where most of the data were missing? Were harms deliberately ignored, or discarded before publication, which they often are in industry-sponsored trials?[87] I find it remarkable, for example, that many people tell me they get muscular pain when they are on statins, which disappear when they stop and come back when they resume the drug, whereas the randomized trials have reported "similar" rates of muscular problems with placebo as with active drugs. I do not believe this. Exposure and reexposure—starting the drug again—is an accepted way of finding out whether drugs cause harms.

The next risk from the CDC: "Vaccine components can on rare occasions cause allergic reactions (immediate hypersensitivity). Manifestations of immediate hypersensitivity range from mild urticaria (hives) and angioedema (swelling beneath the skin) to anaphylaxis." These reactions can be deadly. How often do people die after a flu shot? I have not come across such data.

"In some seasons, the vaccine has been associated with febrile seizures in young children, particularly when given together with 13-valent pneumococcal conjugate vaccine (PCV13) and diphtheria, tetanus and pertussis (DTaP) vaccines." This is highly interesting, considering Aaby's studies (see Chapter 1). We know far too little about the harms caused by simultaneous use of several vaccines and about the harms related to their sequence when not given at the same time. The risk for febrile seizures would have been relevant to know but was not stated.

The next:

> Guillain–Barré Syndrome (GBS) occurs rarely and can cause paralysis. Safety monitoring has not detected a clear link to GBS. However, if there is a risk of GBS from the vaccination, it would be no more than 1 or 2 cases per million people vaccinated. Even though GBS following influenza illness is rare, studies suggest that the risk of developing GBS after having influenza is higher than the potential risk of developing GBS after vaccination.

This looks like a wrong comparison. Few people get influenza whereas it is recommended that all get vaccinated. Thus, the risk of developing GBS could be higher if you get vaccinated than if you don't.

"The vaccine, like other injections, can cause syncope (fainting)." Yes, and in rare cases, this is fatal, e.g., because of head trauma.

* * *

When I googled *most used influenza vaccine*, it seemed that the recombinant vaccine Flublok was the most used one. I looked up the package insert on the FDA website for the quadrivalent version of this vaccine:

> WARNINGS AND PRECAUTIONS. Appropriate medical treatment and supervision must be available to manage possible anaphylactic reactions. If Guillain-Barré syndrome has occurred within 6 weeks of receipt of a prior influenza vaccine, the decision to give Flublok Quadrivalent should be based on careful consideration of potential benefits and risks.
>
> ADVERSE REACTIONS. In adults 18 through 49 years of age, the most common (≥10%) injection-site reactions were tenderness (48%) and pain (37%); the most common (≥10%) solicited systemic adverse reactions were headache (20%), fatigue (17%), myalgia (13%) and arthralgia (10%).

It would have been nice to know what the incidence of these adverse reactions were in the placebo group, particularly the systemic ones, but there were no such data. Tables of adverse reactions had a comparator, but as this was a quadrivalent vaccine from another company, it wasn't helpful.

The Dark Horse in Vaccinations

We are unable to predict, for any vaccine, what the rare but serious harms are. When doctors first alerted their colleagues to the possibility that Pandemrix, one of the influenza vaccines used during the 2009–2010 pandemic, had caused narcolepsy in children and adolescents in Sweden and Finland, their reaction was to ridicule these doctors. It has now been firmly established that Pandemrix can cause narcolepsy, a life-long, seriously debilitating condition with poor treatment options where people suddenly fall asleep, with an onset from about two months after vaccination and up to at least two years later.[88] The manufacturer, GlaxoSmithKline, has settled claims out of court, and the likely mechanism is an autoimmune cross-reaction in people with a particular tissue type between the active component of the vaccine and receptors on brain cells controlling the day rhythm.[89] More than 1,300 people developed narcolepsy from Pandemrix.

Systematic reviews have noted serious deficiencies in safety outcome reporting in published influenza vaccine trials.[90] In 2009, Australia suspended its universal vaccination influenza program for children younger than five years because of a surge in febrile convulsions following vaccination (1 in 110 children).[91] Official inquiries confirmed the vaccine's role. These harms came to light because their incidence was ten times the background rate.

What else do the vaccines cause that we don't know about because the signal is less strong than a factor ten and does not cause alarm in surveillance systems? Influenza vaccines are biologics, and biologic manufacturing is messy, with risks of contamination far in excess of those seen in ordinary drug production.[92] For biologics produced anew each year, these unfortunate events demonstrate that past experience is not necessarily predictive of future vaccine safety.

One might also ask what multiple immunizations lead to? As noted in Chapter 1, studies by Canadian researchers indicated that people who received a seasonal influenza vaccine in 2008 had an increased risk of getting infected with another strain in 2009.[93] They replicated their findings in five different studies. Other researchers have reported that annual influenza vaccination hampers development of CD8 T-cell immunity in children.[94]

At least we now know that influenza vaccines do have important harms. But we do not know all of them, and they may change with the production of altered vaccines. The serious ones are usually very rare, but there are exceptions, as noted earlier.

The Bottom Line of Influenza Vaccination

What should we make out of all this conflicting information? This is not easy, and people will differ as to what they will conclude. What is clear is that we cannot trust the information provided by those whose job it is to care for us. Furthermore, there is no sound basis for the authoritative advice that we should all get vaccinated every year, not only from the cradle to the grave, but even from the womb to the grave.

The CDC admits that repeated influenza vaccination can weaken the immune response to subsequent influenza vaccination and adds that "these findings merit further investigation to understand the immune response to repeat vaccination."[95]

There is convincing research that tells us that there is a price to pay for stimulating the immune system[96] and that vaccines can interact negatively,[97] even when directed against the same virus, as is the case for influenza.[98] Given this knowledge, it seems irresponsible to advise people to get a flu shot every year for their entire life. This is a gigantic, uncontrolled experiment with human beings.

Considering all the hype about flu shots, they are far less popular than you would expect. The differences in usage between the United States and Denmark are huge.[99] In the United States, coverage among children aged 6 months to 17 years is 46%, whereas none get vaccinated in Denmark up to 14 years of age. Coverage among adults in the United States is 45% versus 4% in Denmark between 15 and 64 years. In people aged 65 and above, coverage is 47% in Denmark (this age group is offered free vaccinations by invitation).

When coverage differs so dramatically in two similar countries, it is reasonable to conclude that flu shots are not important.

WHO is far more modest than the CDC.[100] Its highest priority is pregnant women due to their greater susceptibility to severe influenza. It also recommends seasonal vaccination of children aged 6–59 months, elderly, people with specific chronic medical conditions, and healthcare workers. Thus, with few exceptions, WHO leaves out most of the population, those aged 5 to 64 years, which is interesting. I suspect the aggressiveness in the

United States has a lot to do with the extreme degree of unrestrained capitalism that influences US healthcare.

Should all pregnant women get vaccinated? I don't think so. What speaks in favor is that it can be stressful to have an infant with high fever, not knowing what causes it, particularly if you have no experience with childhood infections. You might be worried it could be meningitis or another deadly bacterial infection. It also seems to be safe to get vaccinated during pregnancy.

However, much speaks against vaccinating all pregnant women. The risk of transmitting influenza is only reduced by about 50%; we don't know if vaccination has any effect on outcomes that matter; vaccination can be harmful and may lower the effect of subsequent vaccinations; and the risk of getting influenza is very small and can be lowered by hygienic precautions. Further, there is evidence that nonlive vaccines increase total mortality.[101] I don't think we can recommend vaccination when we don't have reliable data on total mortality and mortality from infections.

The package insert for the often-used recombinant vaccine Flublok Quadrivalent tells us that available data are insufficient to inform vaccine-associated risks in pregnant women. Further, that pregnancy outcomes are being monitored and that healthcare providers are encouraged to report the results to Sanofi Pasteur's vaccination pregnancy registry. No animal studies exist for the quadrivalent vaccine, but a study with the trivalent vaccine did not find evidence of harm to the fetus in rats. We are warned, however, that pregnant women are at increased risk of complications to influenza compared to nonpregnant women and that they may be at increased risk for adverse pregnancy outcomes, including preterm labor.

It is difficult to reduce the risk of a child getting high fever because other viruses than influenza can cause it, and because vaccination does not have an impressive effect. Lived attenuated vaccine reduced the risk of influenza-like illness from 17% to 12%, and inactivated vaccines from 28% to 20%,[102] and the vaccine can give symptoms of illness that might potentially outweigh these small benefits.

At the other end of life, it does not always make sense either to get vaccinated. Some people in nursing homes are in such a bad condition that they will die soon anyway, and some consider that their lives are hardly worth living, e.g., because of serious dementia, urinary and fecal incontinence, and other unpleasant ailments, and say it could be a relief for them to get an infection that will terminate life. We often talk about lives saved in healthcare but virtually never about *which* kind of lives we save. There is an enormous difference between saving an infant's life and a seriously incapacitated person's life. And the effect of vaccinations in older adults on influenza-like illness is small, a reduction in risk from 6% to 3.5%.[103]

My view of doctoring is that people who have survived until old age should preferably be left alone to make their own medical decisions, without intrusions by busybodies equipped with all their guidelines. What is a doctor supposed to do? To inform all the inhabitants in a nursing home every year about influenza and suggest they get vaccinated? Or just do it, which would be against rules for informed consent? What about those who are too demented to understand it, or start screaming or fighting when the doctor approaches them with a needle? Doesn't a doctor tending a nursing home have more important work to do than vaccinating?

Six years ago, two months before his 65th birthday, one of my friends received a letter signed by the mayor for Health and Care. We had a big laugh when we read it:

> It is a great pleasure for me that we, in Copenhagen Municipality, again this
> year can offer free vaccination against influenza to all Copenhageners above
> 65 years of age . . . A vaccination does not give full protection against influ-
> enza, but the vaccine protects most people against serious complications to
> the disease . . . If you have difficulty in moving around outside, you may be
> vaccinated in your own home. If you live in a nursing home, the staff will
> automatically ensure that you will be offered the vaccination.

It is like being invited to mammography screening. The busybodies use a language and a nonexistent familiarity, as if they were inviting you to a private dinner party. We once wrote about this mismatch: "Women like Dorothy . . . have attended without fail for decades."[104] Clearly, not accepting the invitation is a failure, and the omission of Dorothy's surname conveys a sense of familiarity and of belonging to the regular customers' executive club.

It looks like a law of nature that public health messages are always exaggerated. The vaccine does not protect most people against serious complications to the disease; it has not been documented in reliable research that it protects anyone. And now we can see how people in nursing homes will be approached. The staff will ensure not only that they get something to eat, but also that they get an annual injection. What a world this is. I hope I shall never end up in a place where I am no longer my own master. To be free is more important than getting a free injection.

There is a lot else one can do in addition to, or instead of, vaccination. The CDC webpage about vaccine effectiveness ends with this advice: "People should take the same everyday preventive actions to prevent the spread of flu, including covering coughs, washing hands often, and avoiding people who are sick. Antiviral drugs are an important second line of defense to treat the flu."[105]

Stop the nonsense, please. Antiviral drugs are NOT important. They don't seem to work if people take paracetamol (acetaminophen) for their fever, and they have important harms.

Apart from this, it is a very bad idea to use drugs that reduce the fever.[106] An instructive review article noted that the use of antipyretic drugs to diminish fever correlates with a 5% increase in mortality in people with influenza and negatively affects patient outcomes in the intensive care unit.[107]

It is more than a correlation. A lot of research supports the hypothesis that fever is an important response to infection. An increase of 1–4°C (2-7°F) in core body temperature is associated with improved survival and resolution of many infections, and temperatures of 40–41°C (104–106°F) reduce the replication rate of poliovirus in mammalian cells more than 200 times. Fever must have great survival value, as it has been shaped through hundreds of millions of years of natural selection in very different animals. Reptiles, fish, and insects raise their core temperature during infection through behavioral regulation, which leads to their seeking warmer environments despite the higher risk of predation. The survival of the desert iguana *Dipsosaurus dorsalis* is reduced by 75% if prevented from behaviorally raising its core temperature by 2°C (4°F) after infection with the Gram-negative bacterium *Aeromonas hydrophila*.

Coronavirus: The COVID-19 Pandemic

Coronaviruses are best known as causes of the common cold, but there are many variants, and some can cause serious infections. SARS (Severe Acute Respiratory Syndrome) came from bats and emerged in China in 2003.[1] The pandemic lasted only five months, and 774 people died. MERS (Middle East Respiratory Syndrome) emerged in Jordan in 2012 and likely came from dromedary camels. Cases still occur, and by December 2020, the death toll was 919.[2]

A far worse coronavirus pandemic started in Wuhan, China, in November 2019. Like several other virus pandemics, it is suspected to have originated in an animal market, but this is not clear.[3] The disease is caused by severe acute respiratory syndrome coronavirus 2 (SARS-CoV-2) and is called COVID-19 after the year it started.

In the following, months of the year refer to 2020, unless stated otherwise.

Chinese doctor Li Wenliang warned about what looked like a new SARS-like illness in Wuhan in early December 2019 in a group chat with other health professionals.[4] A few days later, he was detained by the police for "spreading false rumours," and they forced him to sign a document admitting that he had "seriously disrupted social order" and breached the law. At least seven other people were similarly disciplined.

Li Wenliang acquired the disease himself and died in early February. His treatment by Chinese authorities sparked outrage across China, and in March, an official report declared that Li had not disrupted public order but was a professional who fought bravely and made sacrifices.[5] The Chinese rulers put the blame on the local police, which added fuel to the anger. On China's Twitter-like Weibo, news of the report had over 160 million views.

On December 31, 2019, Taiwan alerted WHO to the risk of human-to-human transmission of the new virus, but WHO did not pass on the concern to other countries.[6] China has ensured that Taiwan is not a member of WHO, and WHO's cozy relationship with China was criticized, particularly when WHO overly praised China's handling of the coronavirus outbreak despite the fact that China initially covered it up.[7]

This love affair did not last. In January 2021, WHO's director general, Tedros Adhanom Ghebreyesus, said he was "very disappointed" that China, after many months of delay, had still not finalized the permissions for WHO's expert team to enter the country to investigate the origins of COVID-19 in Wuhan.[8]

One year earlier, it took three weeks before China's health ministry confirmed human-to-human transmission, after WHO had said in mid-January that there might be "limited" human-to-human transmission. However, WHO stepped back from this view on the same day. This was the first sign of confusing public announcements, which unfortunately would become a characteristic of this pandemic everywhere.

The disease spread rapidly to the rest of the world, and many measures were introduced to contain the spread of the virus to reduce mortality and to avoid overloading hospitals and intensive care units.

In March, I described the situation as a pandemic of panic.[9] What I missed the most was that the authorities did not heed sufficiently the knowledge researchers already had, and that researchers did not embark on experiments that could tell us what works, what doesn't, and what causes more harm than good. Furthermore, many of the restrictions to ordinary life and other interventions made no sense. We have seen people disinfecting streets, for example, although we know with great certainty that this doesn't work.

Physical Prevention of Disease

Hand hygiene
A 2020 updated systematic review of the randomized trials showed that hand hygiene reduced acute respiratory infections by 16% (risk ratio 0.84, 95% confidence interval 0.82 to 0.86, 44,129 participants), but not influenza-like illness (risk ratio 0.98, 0.85 to 1.13, 32,641 participants).[10]

Face masks

The same review did not find that the use of face masks reduced the occurrence of influenza-like illness (risk ratio 0.99, 0.82 to 1.18, 3507 participants). However, during the first months of the pandemic, the tradition of wearing face masks in public spread from Southeast Asia to the rest of world and became mandatory in many countries.

As the science indicated they didn't work, it is of interest to see how the authorities circumvented this problem.

In the spring, the Danish National Board of Health did not believe that face masks could reduce the risk of becoming infected with COVID-19, and virtually no one wore them.[11] In October, the Board had changed its mind and published a report that justified the use of face masks based on a 2020 review from the *Lancet*. This review is unreliable[12] and has been seriously criticized.[13] It was a review of observational studies, and the apparent effect is likely due to the fact that people who voluntarily choose to wear face masks are more careful with hand hygiene and with keeping their distance from other people than people who do not wear face masks—a classic error in observational research called *confounding*.

A problem with health authorities in all countries is that they do not distinguish clearly between science and politics. The Board wrote that randomized trials—where only half of the people wear face masks—are most reliable and cited the updated systematic review of such trials that did not find an effect of face masks. But then came the trick: the Board argued that as there were no results from randomized trials addressing *coronavirus*, observational studies were the best to say something about the effect of face masks. This is not a valid argument. Influenza viruses and coronaviruses spread in the same way, and they have the same size, about 100 nm. The results of randomized trials with face masks for influenza-like viruses therefore also apply to coronavirus.

Three weeks after the Board's report, a Danish randomized trial of face masks in 6,024 people was published.[14] Infection with SARS-CoV-2 occurred in 42 participants asked to wear masks (1.8%) and in 53 control participants (2.1%), a difference of 0.3% (-0.4% to 1.2%, p = 0.33). The researchers had offered the Board to look at the manuscript before it published its own report, which the Board declined. Obviously, politics was more important than science.

It can be argued that face masks *might* work, as there was a nonsignificant tendency toward fewer coronavirus infections when people wore them, and that they should therefore be used, as they cause no harm.

I do not agree with this. First, the risk ratio for preventing influenza-like illness was 0.99, and if the Danish trial results are added to this in a meta-analysis, the risk ratio becomes 0.96 (0.81 to 1.13, p = 0.63), or almost the same. This does not give much hope. Second, face masks cause harm. They are uncomfortable to wear, can cause highly irritating itching in the nose and pimples, and can cause impaired vision if you wear glasses and it is cold. They might also give the wearers a false sense of security so that they come too close to other customers in shops. In contrast to face masks, keeping distance works: if people do not come close to one another, they do not get infected.

We should not mandate whole populations to look like bank robbers for months or years when the science indicates that they don't work. Furthermore, there is no logic in the requirements. In Denmark, children below 12 years of age do not need to wear face masks, even though this age group likely spreads more infections than others.

Finally, I have not met a single person who uses face masks correctly. People use the same mask over and over, sometimes for weeks. According to guidelines, it is not even allowed to put it temporarily in your pocket in order to reuse it for the next shop on your shopping route. Very few people are aware of this. Face masks have become a symbol of belonging to the crowd, of feeling good, rather than a help.

It should be voluntary to wear face masks. People who are concerned about coronavirus or who think they might have become infected could wear them if they want to. People can also choose to wear them when they visit old people and others who have a considerable risk of dying if infected. My family doesn't do that when we visit our frail relatives. We keep our distance, which is what matters.

Keeping distance

Peter Aaby's studies have taught us that the infectious dose of a virus is an important determinant for whether we will survive or die (see Chapter 2). If the dose is too high, the immune system cannot mount an effective response before it is too late.

This is an important reason why so many people died in overcrowded hospitals in northern Italy and in China, where secret recordings showed corpses lying on the hospital floor and staff that was too busy to remove them while the only protection they had was face masks.

Forbidding gatherings of people is highly effective. The pandemic hit Bergamo in Italy very hard because one-third of the city watched a

Champions League football match in Milano in February and celebrated the local team's win deep into the night.[15]

There are no randomized trials of physical distancing.[16] Despite the wide range of social-distancing policies adopted in various countries, the decline in the number of deaths in countries that did not apply effective measures from the start of the pandemic has been remarkably similar.[17] This suggests that, as long as social distancing is implemented, what remains is an inherent element of the epidemic's dynamic that is the same everywhere.

In Italy, the military was commanded to patrol the streets, and people were only allowed to leave the house once a day for shopping or going to a pharmacy or walking the dog (close to the house only), which led people to borrow dogs to get a little fresh air. In Spain, people were not allowed to run in the forest, and everyone leaving the house had to wear face masks.

I joked a lot about the absurdities and was surprised to experience that all my jokes but one came true. When the Danish government announced in March that only gatherings of two people would be allowed[18] (the proposal was not carried through, though), I said that our prime minister would soon only allow one person at a time in double beds, as it was important to keep the social distance at 2 meters.

Even my most bizarre joke came true. After having seen a photo of a couple in a canoe in Spain, totally alone but wearing face masks, I joked that I looked forward to seeing a photo of a couple making love naked while wearing face masks. In September, Canada's chief medical officer advised people to skip kissing and consider wearing a mask when having sex, adding that going solo was safest: "The lowest risk sexual activity during COVID-19 involves yourself alone."[19] Well, if you only masturbate, you won't get sexually transmitted diseases, either. And if you don't get out of bed, you won't get COVID-19. But your life will be over.

Lockdowns

I have not seen any country formulating a clear lockdown strategy based on science or an exit strategy. Many countries have run a zigzag course between closing and opening; ministers have switched back and forth between alarm and reassurance; and drastic lockdowns have been introduced based on highly doubtful research that used modeling, which can give you virtually any result you want depending on what you put into the model.

Kindergartens, schools, universities, shopping centers, and restaurants were closed; meetings were canceled; football matches were cancelled; and when they came back it was without spectators.

A systematic review found that school closures did not contribute to the control of the SARS epidemic in China, Hong Kong, and Singapore.[20] If children are sent home to be looked after by their grandparents because their parents are at work, it could bode disaster for the grandparents. In the United Kingdom, the median age of those who die is 83.[21]

I wonder why we have not seen randomized trials of school closure. In Norway, researchers attempted to do such a study, but the government officials were unwilling to keep schools open.[22] Only two months later, when the virus waned, they refused to keep schools closed, and Norwegian TV shot the messenger: "Crazy researcher wants to experiment with children."

In America, the priorities were different. In many large American cities, bars were open while schools were closed.

Many of the restrictions were illogical. In Denmark, golf courses were closed, which led to the absurdity that you were allowed to walk on the fairways as long as you did not look like a golfer. Tennis courts were closed, although gatherings of four people were not forbidden. Even outdoor running clubs closed.

The big issue about avoiding crowding is that we do not know where to stop. When do lockdowns become more harmful than beneficial? I shall explain later that we came far out on the harmful side a long time ago and have continued down that path.

Closing borders
We do not know if it helps to close borders, but we do know that it is immensely harmful and disrupts people's lives substantially.

In Denmark, we closed our borders with Germany and Sweden when we had more coronavirus than they had. I joked that, using the same logic, we might as well have closed the island of Fyn, in the middle of Denmark, which is easy, as there is a bridge on each side that can be blocked by the military. Eight months later, our government did for a while close all travel across municipal boundaries in Northern Denmark, even for people who worked outdoors after a coronavirus mutation in mink had been found up there.

Most countries have introduced total or partial travel restrictions. In December, at long last, we saw some sanity coming along when the European Centre for Disease Prevention and Control and the European Union Aviation Safety Agency issued new guidelines.[23] They realized that, because COVID-19 was everywhere, imported cases accounted for a very small proportion of all detected cases and were unlikely to significantly increase the rate of transmission. As the prevalence of the disease in travelers was likely lower than the prevalence in the general population or among contacts of confirmed cases, travelers should not be considered a high-risk population, and EU member states should facilitate swift transit. Furthermore, quarantine or systematic testing for SARS-CoV-2 of air travelers was not recommended.

However, the same month, when a mutant in the UK with 50–70% higher infectivity had been found, border restrictions were immediately reintroduced. Visitors from the United Kingdom were banned, and Danes living in the United Kingdom were strongly discouraged from visiting Denmark.

This is unbearable. Panic, panic, panic, with little justification but causing huge harm. Will this ever stop?

In November, the Australian airline Qantas announced compulsory vaccination for all passengers on international flights. This human rights violation was immediately grounded by the CEO of the International Air Transport Association (IATA), who said that the industry would die if it were to wait for the deployment of vaccines.[24] The airline industry has been projected to lose US$157 billion.

Several countries require a negative coronavirus test taken within the last three days before leaving the airport. As screening healthy people will yield many false positives (see below), you might lose both your holiday and your money for no good reason. There are no randomized trials of the effect of screening at departure or entry ports.[25]

Quarantine

It would seem prudent to ask infected people to stay in their homes so that they do not infect people in the community, and this has been recommended in almost all countries. But Aaby's studies have taught us that it is not a good idea. The index person—the one who gets infected in the community—will often have a good prognosis because of low viral load. When that person is ordered to stay at home, secondarily infected people in the household will have a considerably higher risk of dying because the infectious dose will be much higher for people living closely together who are exposed to repeated transmission from a person in whom the virus has multiplied. Aaby has shown that, in Guinea-Bissau, the mortality for secondary cases of measles in the home was 3–4 times higher than for the index case.[26]

There is a quasi-cluster-randomized trial that studied the effect of quarantine.[27] During the 2009–2010 influenza pandemic, fewer company employees in Japan contracted influenza when people who had a household member with influenza-like illness symptoms were asked to stay at home compared with employees in the control group, 2.75% versus 3.18%, hazard ratio 0.80 (0.66 to 0.97). However, those asked to stay at home with their infected family member were twice as likely to become infected.

Air-conditioning
In the United States, air-conditioning is running constantly in hotels and elsewhere, and often to excess. Whether it is warm or cold outside or inside is immaterial. I have often frozen bitterly at American meetings while it was warm summer outside. I have not reviewed the research, but we know that lethal lung infections have spread this way, e.g., with Legionella, which is a bacterium.

The Best and the Worst Countries

As explained, the authorities should not send infected people home but isolate them in quarantine centers, e.g., in sports arenas, conference halls, or hotel rooms, until they are no longer infectious. This has been the strategy in China and in a few other countries in Southeast Asia. In most countries, there are strong cultural barriers against such a drastic measure.

Overcrowding was avoided in South Korea, where only severely ill patients were allowed to get to the hospital.[28] South Korea and Taiwan used aggressive early contact tracing and isolated the cases,[29] which meant that people could go to the gym and eat at a restaurant, while in most other countries, virtually everything was closed.

Taiwan was well prepared. During the 2003 SARS epidemic, 73 people died in Taiwan, and since then, many city dwellers have worn face masks voluntarily to protect against respiratory viruses. When Taiwan learned about a new disease in Wuhan, on December 31, 2019, the country reacted immediately, on the very first day.[30] There was strict surveillance of those infected who were given a mobile phone with an app that constantly reported where they were. Isolation lasted two weeks, and the punishment for breaking it was harsh: a patient who left the hotel room for only eight seconds received a fine corresponding to 2,800 Euros.[31]

One year later, when most of the world was locked down, people in Taiwan could go to concerts with thousands of people and to restaurants. They have now made it mandatory to wear face masks in schools, restaurants, and at cultural arrangements, but this was not because more people became infected, but because rates went up in other countries. For the same reason, Taiwan employs a two-week quarantine for people coming from abroad.

Taiwan is close to China, and about 850,000 Taiwanese live there. American experts therefore predicted a high mortality rate, but it is one of the lowest in the world. Only 7 patients have died from COVID-19, which is 0.3 per million inhabitants.[32] As of December 20, 974 per million have died in the United States, which is over 3,000 times as many.[33] In the table below, I have shown data from 24 countries to illustrate by how much COVID-19 mortality rates differ between countries and parts of the world one year into the pandemic.[34]

It can be difficult to know if a person died from, or only with, COVID-19, and reporting standards vary between countries. Furthermore, the virus mutates. However, the differences between mortality rates per million people are so large that they dwarf any methodological concerns:

Belgium	1,597	Germany	315
Italy	1,133	Denmark	176
Spain	1,046	Finland	88
UK	986	Iceland	82
USA	974	Norway	74
France	925	Australia	35
Brazil	874	Japan	22
Sweden	789	S. Korea	13
Netherlands	610	Singapore	5
South Africa	411	New Zealand	5
Canada	373	Taiwan	0.3
Russia	345	Tanzania	0.3

In Southeast Asia, there have been few deaths. The official mortality rate for China is 3, but we cannot trust mortality data from this country where all information is tightly controlled by the one-party leaders and where dissidents are brutally punished.

There have also been relatively few deaths in the five Nordic countries, with Sweden as a marked exception. Sweden has a mortality rate about ten times as large as Norway and Finland, which are as sparsely populated as Sweden. In contrast to Sweden, there has been no excess mortality in Finland, Denmark, and Norway.[35]

Denmark has a population density that is 8–10 times higher than in the other countries, and it reacted quite late to the pandemic. On February 23, the Danish National Board of Health maintained that there was a very low risk that the virus would spread to Denmark. However, only two weeks later, the government encouraged cancellations of events with more than 1,000 participants,[36] and after another week, we had our first COVID-19 deaths, and the government panicked.

These facts can perhaps explain why the mortality rate in Denmark is twice as large as in Norway and Finland. The official narrative is that we have been very good at tackling the pandemic, but this can be discussed. Our contact tracing has worked poorly. We have focused on social distancing, hand hygiene, and lockdown. When this was not enough, it became obligatory from August to wear face masks while in public transportation and also two months later in shops.

Why did Sweden do so poorly, and why did the gap widen throughout 2020? In April, there were 2.2 times more COVID-19 deaths per million in Sweden than in Denmark, and in December, there were 4.5 times as many.

Sweden remained an open society that did not close institutions or restaurants, and it took until mid-March before they canceled events with 500 or more participants.[37] At the same time, Denmark made all gatherings of more than 10 people illegal, warning that law offenders would be fined by the police.[38]

One of the arguments for keeping the Swedish society open was to establish herd immunity by allowing the virus to spread, so that future waves of infection would be milder. Since young people tolerate the infection very well and very few below 50 years of age die from the infection, unless they have serious comorbidity or are extremely overweight, this idea seemed reasonable. However, Sweden forgot to protect its most vulnerable citizens, e.g., those living in nursing homes, sufficiently, and after a year, Sweden realized its experiment had failed and tightened its regulations.

* * *

The United States, the United Kingdom, Brazil, and Russia failed miserably. An important reason for this is that they were all run by populist male leaders who cast themselves as anti-elite and anti-establishment.[39] Such leaders tend to reject scientific advice, propagate lies and fake news, promote conspiracy theories, and claim they have a kind of greatness and common-sense wisdom that experts lack.

In the United States, President Trump said 40 times that the virus would disappear[40] "like a miracle,"[41] suggested that injecting a disinfectant could cure the illness,[42] and proposed irradiating patients' bodies with UV light either from the outside or the inside.[43]

Brazilian president Bolsonaro called COVID-19 a "small cold" and tried to remove statistics on the Internet that told a different story about infections and deaths, which the supreme court prevented him from accomplishing.[44]

In 2019, two months before the first case of COVID-19 appeared, a new scorecard was published, the Global Health Security Index, which ranked countries on how prepared they were to tackle a serious infectious disease outbreak.[45] The United States came first, and the United Kingdom was second.

The scorecard did not account for the political context, and the reality was the exact opposite. It has been estimated that the United States comes first, and the United Kingdom second in terms of excess deaths (deaths that might have been avoided).[46] Even before COVID-19 hit, President Trump and Prime Minister Johnson had devalued the importance of public health investment and degraded their national pandemic preparedness capabilities.

On January 23, WHO told all countries that they were at risk of a COVID-19 epidemic, advising them to get prepared to track and isolate cases. Both countries ignored the warning. In April, England's deputy chief medical officer argued that track and trace was not needed, and Trump encouraged people to defy orders to work from home. In November, *BMJ*'s editor asked: "How has testing become an end in itself, divorced (in the UK at least) from a functioning system of contact tracing and isolation? Why this refusal to abandon failed centralised and commercial approaches and instead to properly fund local public sector systems of find, test, trace, isolate, and support? Is it ideology, ignorance, incompetence, or vested interest?"[47]

The systematic failings had huge consequences. The United Kingdom and the United States introduced lockdowns very late, and with insufficient capability to test people, trace contacts, and isolate them. New York had plenty of time to prepare for the pandemic, as it was hit two months later than Taiwan.

Populist leaders' anti-expertise response and nonsense is deadly.[48] So far, there have been over 400,000 deaths in the United States and in the

United Kingdom. If they had had the same mortality rate as Taiwan, only 120 people would have died.

* * *

With only 5 deaths per million, New Zealand is a success story. While avoiding totalitarian abuses such as those seen in China, both Taiwan and New Zealand have had a clear and consequential approach to the pandemic. They are democracies with well-functioning public sectors and healthcare, but their approaches have been different. Taiwan had open schools with universal use of face masks constructed specifically for children, while New Zealand did the opposite. Such experiences do not make it easier when we try to find out what is best, but at the very least, it seems that it is not necessary to do both, which is what almost all countries do.

Is the New Coronavirus Worse than Influenza Viruses?

Considering all the deaths, it seems foolish to ask this question, but if we want to understand what is happening, it is essential to distinguish between the inherent biological properties of viruses and the circumstances under which they operate.

The same virus can kill relatively few people, or it can become very deadly if there is overcrowding and it hits a nonimmune population. In the Faroe Islands, measles had not prevailed since 1781 when it broke out 65 years later, in 1846.[49] During the epidemic, 78% were attacked and the case fatality rate was 2.8%, which is over 10 times higher than the usual rate of about 0.2%.

The information from the authorities has been confusing. WHO's director general announced in March that COVID-19 was *less* contagious than influenza based on the data they had seen so far,[50] but five weeks later he said that COVID-19 spreads fast.

This was the key argument for the lockdowns and other physical measures. But whenever I asked for evidence that the coronavirus is much more contagious than the influenza virus, I did not get convincing replies. The transmission rates seem to be similar.[51] Early on, there was an outbreak on the Diamond Princess Cruise ship where an entire, closed population of quarantined passengers and crew were tested for the virus.[52] The infection rate was only 19% even though people had crowded in bars, at buffets, and on the dance floor.

Another example is when my wife sat close to a junior doctor while tutoring him for over an hour at the hospital where she works. He developed symptoms and tested positive the next day, but although he had been close to numerous people at the department, not a single person was infected. He only infected his daughter.

Such experiences prove that the new coronavirus is not in league with measles or smallpox, which are highly infectious, but behaves more like influenza. This is still the case, even after a mutant with greater infectivity was located in the United Kingdom.

The most important argument has been that the coronavirus is much more deadly than influenza. In March, WHO's director general stated: "Globally, about 3.4% of reported COVID-19 cases have died. By comparison, seasonal flu generally kills far fewer than 1% of those infected."[53]

WHO did not take into account that the denominator—the number of infected people—was vastly underestimated. Its mortality estimate for COVID-19 was exaggerated by a factor of more than 10. The result of the misleading announcement was to cause horror and more panic than there already was.[54]

The best evidence we have suggests the death risks are similar. As the risk of dying depends on the infectious dose, which is higher in settings with overcrowding, we can only estimate death rates approximately. As already noted, in outbreaks of measles, a common estimate is 0.2%, but it can be 50 times higher. In Vienna, at the beginning of the twentieth century, the mortality was 11% among the poorest and 0.6% among the richest (see Chapter 3). We have also seen a strong social gradient for COVID-19 deaths, likely because the poor have small living spaces.

In Denmark, blood donors were tested for coronavirus antibodies in April, and the estimated mortality rate was 0.16%,[55] the same as for measles.

The preliminary case fatality rate on the Diamond Princess Cruise ship was 1.0%,[56] but this was a largely elderly population in a crowded environment, and projecting the mortality rate onto the age structure of the US population, the death rate would be 0.13%.[57] This estimate was based on only seven deaths, but it was similar to the Danish estimate.

A more recent estimate comes from a systematic review that included 82 single estimates.[58] The median COVID-19 infection fatality rate was 0.27%, and it was only 0.05% for people below 70 years of age. Both rates are likely exaggerated, as most of the studies were from locations with higher mortality rates than average. The inferred median infection fatality rate in locations with a COVID-19 mortality rate lower than average was only 0.09%.

For influenza, there are huge variations in reported case-fatality rates. A graph in a systematic review showed a median of 1% for laboratory-confirmed influenza during the 2009 influenza pandemic and the following years,[59] but this is likely also exaggerated.

As noted, the median age of those who die from coronavirus is over 80, and most of them had important comorbidity like heart or lung disease. In Italy, 99% of those who died had at least one comorbidity.[60] These are also the type of people who die during influenza epidemics. In Lombardy, many factors contributed to the high death rates. The hospitals were overcrowded; they admitted even mild cases; the staff did not have much protection initially; and there was a lack of personal hygiene. Furthermore, the Italian population is relatively old; people smoke more; generations live close together; and there is a lovely tradition of hugging and kissing anyone.

When I debate with people, they have great difficulty accepting that the new coronavirus might not be worse than influenza viruses in terms of contagiousness and case fatality rate. A typical argument is: "I have seen many patients die in my intensive care unit from COVID-19 but never anyone dying from influenza." I think this can be understood by comparing with measles epidemics. Influenza epidemics never hit a nonimmune population. Furthermore, when millions get infected, many die, even when the infection fatality rate is low. People's clinical experience is often misleading; we need to look at the numbers in the nominator and denominator.

Drugs

Corticosteroids seem to be effective for patients with acute respiratory distress syndrome and therefore also for COVID-19 patients in intensive care units.[61]

Other drugs touted for treating COVID-19 have been a big disappointment.[62] Hydroxychloroquine was promoted by French researcher Didier Raoult based on a small, totally flawed study he did with no control group, and it was touted by US President Trump and his personal lawyer, former New York City mayor Rudolph Giuliani, who claimed 100% efficacy.[63] Trump announced that he would send 2 million doses of hydroxychloroquine to Brazil,[64] and the FDA spinelessly buckled to the political pressure and issued an emergency authorization giving doctors a green light to prescribe it,[65] which the agency later rescinded. Hydroxychloroquine does not work and has fatal harms, but usage in the US increased 525%.[66] The large WHO Solidarity trial found that hydroxychloroquine increased mortality, rate ratio 1.19 (0.89 to 1.59, p = 0.23; 104/947 vs 84/906 patients died), and it also increased the initiation of ventilation and hospital stay.[67]

Remdesivir (Veklury) was hyped to the extreme, and its history is very dirty. Two weeks before Anthony S. Fauci announced at a White House press conference in April that the drug would be the new "standard of care," the investigators of a trial partly funded by the US National Institutes of Health (NIH) changed the primary outcome, which was the death rate, and replaced it with the time it took patients to recover.[68] For obvious reasons, such outcome switching shortly before a trial is published is considered scientific misconduct.

Fauci's announcement coincided with the publication of a Chinese placebo-controlled trial the same day in the *Lancet* that did not find any positive effects of remdesivir. What the White House did is called science by press release, which is a violation of accepted scientific principles. Academic institutions also distributed dramatic results in press releases before anyone could check if the research was valid. The coronavirus epidemic has not only killed people, but also our ethical norms.

It took another three weeks before the preliminary results of the trial were published in . . . guess where . . . the *New England Journal of Medicine* of course, as it was a US trial.[69] It could also have been in the *Lancet*, another key journal for irreproducible industry results that are highly enriching, both for the journal and for big pharma. The preliminary report was published on the journal's website and cannot be found on PubMed, which is puzzling. All Internet searches lead to the final report, which was published in October, six months later.

When the preliminary results were published, I explained that we did not know what the true value of remdesivir was.[70] Two of the coauthors, Danish professors Jens Lundgren and Thomas Benfield, who have constantly been in the TV news during the pandemic, touted remdesivir as a miracle drug. Even though it had no significant effect on mortality, Lundgren said that if the drug was given at the right time, it could reduce mortality by about 80%. Benfield called the results "totally unbelievable," which indeed they were.

When Benfield was interviewed about the trial for the *Journal of the Danish Medical Association*, he declared as a conflict of interest that he was an investigator in the trial. When I looked up his conflicts of interest on the homepage of the *New England Journal of Medicine*, it turned out that he had received grants and personal fees from Gilead (the manufacturer of remdesivir); "unrestricted grants" (a euphemism for corruption[71]) from Pfizer,

Novo Nordisk Foundation, Simonsen Foundation, and GSK; personal fees from GSK, Pfizer, Boehringer Ingelheim, and MSD; and grants from the Lundbeck Foundation. This is a bit more than just being an investigator in a trial sponsored by public funds and governments.

On October 15, the results from the much bigger WHO Solidarity trial were published. The rate ratio for mortality was 0.95 (0.81 to 1.11, p = 0.50; 301 vs 303 patients died).[72] Combining the data from all four remdesivir trials, the rate ratio was 0.91 (0.79 to 1.05).[73] Like hydroxychloroquine, remdesivir increased the initiation of ventilation and hospital stay. It was also puzzling that the Chinese remdesivir trial had not found any reduction in viral load, without which it is difficult to imagine that the drug could work.[74]

The Solidarity trial was exemplary, but it was unduly attacked by Gilead the same day: "It is unclear if any conclusive findings can be drawn from the study results." The whole affair was so ugly that *Science* called it "The 'very, very bad look' of remdesivir" in its headline.[75]

On October 8, Gilead entered an agreement to supply the European Union with remdesivir, a deal for $1.2 billion. Gilead received the WHO data already on September 23 but did not reveal its results to the European Commission, which only learned about them from the European Medicines Agency the day after they had signed the agreement with Gilead.

In May, the FDA granted remdesivir an emergency use authorization, which became broadened in August. In its review from October 21 that granted remdesivir full approval, the FDA only included data from three trials: the NIH study and two Gilead-sponsored trials. The FDA ignored the Solidarity data as well as the findings from the placebo-controlled trial in China. Understandably, this scandalous, harmful, and totally unscientific approach of a major drug regulator infuriated the Solidarity team.

Gilead locked EU members into a handsome price of about $2400 for a full course of its ineffective drug. In the United States, the waste was huge. In the third quarter of 2020, Gilead sold $873 million of remdesivir, almost entirely in the United States, as the Trump administration secured almost all of Gilead's supply during the quarter.[76] About half of the patients hospitalized in the United States were treated with the drug.

Drug regulators rarely admit even their most horrible failures. WHO recommends against using remdesivir, but EMA approved it in July, and although the agency announced in November that it would evaluate the data from the Solidarity trial,[77] nothing has happened so far. It should not be that difficult. It takes less than an hour to read the trial report.

Vaccines

Vaccines were developed with a stunning speed, never seen before in healthcare. It only took one year from the outbreak in Wuhan until the first three vaccines had received approval for emergency use and interim analyses of large trials had been published, in the *Lancet*[78] and *New England Journal of Medicine*.[79]

This was thanks to our governments that invested a huge amount of money in the research, after which big drug companies commercialized the vaccines and did the randomized trials.

The University of Oxford-AstraZeneca vaccine uses a replication-deficient chimpanzee adenoviral vector containing the spike protein of the coronavirus.[80] The BioNTech-Pfizer and the NIH-Moderna vaccines are messenger RNA vaccines that instruct cells to manufacture a protein that looks like the spike protein of the coronavirus. About storage, the published Pfizer trial report only says that "very cold temperatures are required."[81] According to an FDA briefing document, "very cold" means between -60°C and -80°C,[82] which is indeed very, very cold. The two other vaccines can be stored in a refrigerator.

Only one of 50 severe cases of COVID-19 occurred in the vaccine groups, and two COVID-19 deaths occurred in the control groups. The data in the individual trials were 0 vs. 10 (one death),[83] 1 vs. 9 ,[84] and 0 vs. 30 (one death).[85]

There were 5 vs. 10 deaths not related to COVID-19 in the trials (cardiovascular causes 6, unknown 2, and road traffic accident, trauma, homicide, suicide, fungal pneumonia, intraabdominal perforation, and leukemia 1 each).

These results are highly encouraging. We do not know yet if the vaccines reduce mortality, but it is very likely, and we will hopefully soon get the answer now that many millions of people get vaccinated.

As death is the most important and also the only unbiased outcome, it is surprising that the primary outcome for the vaccine trials was confirmed COVID-19 infection, which in most cases is a banal infection like the common cold.

All three trial reports are confusing to read, and essential data on harms are missing. I needed to do cumbersome detective work that included reading supplements, protocols, and FDA reports. This should not have been necessary.

None of the trial reports defined what they meant by a serious adverse event. According to the FDA, it means that the outcome is death;

life-threatening; hospitalization (initial or prolonged); disability or permanent damage; congenital anomaly/birth defect; intervention to prevent permanent impairment or damage (devices); or jeopardy of the patient and
medical or surgical intervention to prevent one of the other outcomes, e.g.,
allergic bronchospasm.

None of the efficacy trials was adequately blinded, as the staff admin-
istering the vaccine knew its identity. This fragile arrangement means that
some of the patients or investigators might have been aware if vaccine or
control had been given.

The Oxford-AstraZeneca vaccine

The published report describes four trials.[86] Only two contributed to the
efficacy analyses. In one, 3,744 participants received the vaccine and 3,804
a meningococcal vaccine; in the other, these numbers were 2,063 vs. 2,025,
but the second dose was not the meningococcal vaccine, but a saline placebo.

All four trials contributed data to the safety analyses. In one of the
additional trials, 534 vs. 533 participants received the vaccine or a meningococcal vaccine; in the other, 1,008 vs. 1,005 received the vaccine or a saline
placebo. Only the safety trial with a saline placebo was double blind.

The participants were asked to contact the study site if they experienced
symptoms associated with COVID-19 and received regular reminders to do
so. If they had any one of the following—fever of at least 37.8°C, cough,
shortness of breath, and loss of smell or taste—a swab was taken for a PCR
test (polymerase chain reaction test, also called a nucleic acid amplification
test, NAAT).

Vaccine efficacy was 70% (30 of 5,807 vs. 101 of 5,829 were infected
and had symptoms). In participants who received two full vaccine doses,
vaccine efficacy was 62%, whereas it was 90% in those who received a low
dose plus a full dose ($p = 0.01$ for the difference). This could be a chance
finding.

There are no data on numbers of patients with severe adverse events
(those preventing daily activity), only on the numbers of such events, 84
vs. 91 (175 in total, but only 168 patients had events). Thus, the vaccine did
not increase severe adverse events, but the trials were not adequate to study
vaccine harms, as 86% of the patients in the control groups received another
vaccine and not placebo.

Serious adverse events occurred in 79 patients receiving the vaccine and
in 89 receiving the meningococcal vaccine or saline. A supplement describes
all these events.

Three of the authors were employees of AstraZeneca; one reported personal fees from the company and one nonfinancial support. Three were inventors of patents related to the vaccine; one had received personal fees; and four had other conflicts of interest. Seventy of the 82 authors (85%) had not declared any conflicts of interest.

The BioNTech-Pfizer vaccine

Pfizer did not tell its readers that the blinding of the trial was compromised.[87] The trial report only mentioned—and only in the abstract—that the study was "observer-blinded." As the control was a saline placebo, one would expect the vials to be identical in appearance. A supplement contained Pfizer's protocol, which explained that "the physical appearance of the investigational vaccine candidates and the placebo may differ."

Another reason why this trial cannot have been effectively blinded is that the vaccine causes substantial harms compared to placebo. This was also obscured in the article. The reporting of adverse events took up 2.5 pages, but they were shown in bar charts and split into subgroups after age, first or second vaccine dose, and type of event, which is immensely irritating and unhelpful. A supplement showed that any adverse event occurred in 26.7% vs. 12.2% of the patients. Thus, the number needed to vaccinate to harm one patient was only 7 (the inverse of the risk difference).

There were other problems. FDA's briefing document showed that 311 vs. 60 patients were excluded from the efficacy analyses because of "other important protocol deviations"[88] ($p = 2 \times 10^{-42}$ for this huge difference, my calculation). There was no explanation why many more patients had been excluded from the vaccine group than from the placebo group.

Vaccine efficacy was 95% (8 of 21,720 vs. 162 of 21,728 patients became infected). This assessment might have been biased. According to FDA criteria, confirmed COVID-19 was defined as a positive PCR test and the presence of at least one of the following symptoms: fever, new or increased cough, new or increased shortness of breath, chills, new or increased muscle pain, new loss of taste or smell, sore throat, diarrhea, or vomiting.

The problem with this is that the vaccine causes some of the same symptoms. Pfizer's trial protocol contains a remarkable statement: "During the 7 days following each vaccination, potential COVID-19 symptoms that overlap with specific systemic events (i.e., fever, chills, new or increased muscle pain, diarrhea, vomiting) should not trigger a potential COVID-19 illness visit unless, in the investigator's opinion, the clinical picture is more indicative of a possible COVID-19 illness than vaccine reactogenicity. If, in the investigator's opinion, the symptoms are considered more likely to be vaccine reactogenicity, but a participant is required to demonstrate that they are SARS-CoV-2–negative, a local SARS-CoV-2 test may be performed."[89]

The investigators were discouraged from finding out if patients with symptoms were infected unless the patient needed a negative test, e.g., to be allowed to go to work. According to the FDA report, suspected COVID-19 cases that occurred within 7 days after any vaccination were 409 in the vaccine group vs. only 287 in the placebo group ($p = 3 \times 10^{-6}$, my calculation), and patients over 55 years of age used antipyretics or pain medications more commonly after the vaccine than after placebo; the difference in usage was 8% after the first dose and 28% after the second.[90] Pfizer's inappropriate instructions to investigators and the greater use of drugs that could mask symptoms of COVID-19 mean that the true effect of the vaccine could be less than what was reported but, judged by the incidence curves of confirmed cases, this was likely a minor problem.

It was more concerning that the protocol stated that "Three blinded case reviewers (medically qualified Pfizer staff members) will review all potential COVID-19 illness events."

A secondary outcome was severe COVID-19 defined by the FDA as confirmed infection plus clinical signs at rest with one of the following additional features: clinical signs at rest that are indicative of severe systemic illness; respiratory failure; evidence of shock; significant acute renal, hepatic, or neurologic dysfunction; admission to an intensive care unit; or death. "Clinical signs at rest that are indicative of severe systemic illness" is left entirely to the clinician's discretion. This is subjective, and when the blinding is not impeccable, it can introduce bias, as the clinician could be more inclined to make this decision for patients on placebo.

Pfizer's article was obscure for severe adverse events. A supplement showed that 240 patients (1.1%) had severe adverse events on the vaccine versus 139 (0.6%) on placebo. Pfizer did not provide a p-value, but $p = 2 \times 10^{-7}$. The number needed to vaccinate to harm one patient severely was therefore 200. As severe harm "prevents daily activity," one in 200 became temporarily incapacitated when they received the vaccine who would have been fine without the vaccine. Pfizer's article was seriously misleading, as it said nothing about this, only that "The safety profile of BNT162b2 was characterized by short-term, mild-to-moderate pain at the injection site, fatigue, and headache."

In the FDA report, severe adverse events were detailed in a so-called reactogenicity subset of patients.[91] In patients 18 to 55 years of age, the differences between vaccine and placebo after the second dose were 3.9% for severe fatigue, 2.5% for severe headache, and 2.1% for severe muscle pain. Even though the median duration of these symptoms was only one day, the FDA report told a totally different story to the journal publication. The number needed to harm was only 26 for severe fatigue.

The difference in solicited systemic adverse events (all severities) within 7 days after the first vaccine dose was 12%, which increased to 36% (70% vs. 34%) after the second dose. Thus, the number needed to harm was only 3 after the second dose.

Serious adverse events were extremely poorly reported. Apart from deaths, the trial report mentioned only those considered related to the vaccine: none in the placebo group and four in the vaccine group, shoulder injury related to vaccine administration, right axillary lymphadenopathy, paroxysmal ventricular arrhythmia, and right leg paraesthesia.

The Discussion noted that "The incidence of serious adverse events was similar in the vaccine and placebo groups (0.6% and 0.5%, respectively)." That was all. No numbers. The FDA report revealed that the numbers were 126 vs. 111 (p = 0.33, my calculation). I could not see anywhere what these 237 serious adverse events were about.

The most important numbers are ALL patients with serious adverse events, not just a tiny fraction of them (2%) that investigators, most of whom were on Pfizer's payroll, opined were related to the drugs. A supplement showed that 18 of the 29 authors of the trial report had received personal fees from Pfizer and 15 held stock in Pfizer. Only 8 authors (28%) had not declared any conflicts of interest. We do not expect authors who are so conflicted to report honestly on the harms they found, which they didn't do, either.

The FDA report acknowledged that more patients "would be needed to confirm efficacy of the vaccine against mortality. However, non-COVID vaccines (e.g., influenza) that are efficacious against disease have also been shown to prevent disease-associated death."[92] This is blatantly false (see Chapter 4). Drug regulators should stick to the facts and refrain from wishful thinking. We have enough of this from the drug companies.

The NIH-Moderna vaccine
This trial was described in the abstract as an "observer-blinded, placebo-controlled trial," which is somewhat contradictory, as we use placebos to blind trials, not only to blind observers.[93] However, even though the control was

a saline placebo, the pharmacists and vaccine administrators were aware of treatment assignments.

Vaccine efficacy was 94.1% (11 of 14,134 vs. 185 of 14,073 were infected and had symptoms). However, as 15,210 were randomized to each group, 1,076 vs. 1,147 patients were missing. It was very difficult to find out what had happened, but it seems that the analysis only included patients in "the per-protocol population," with "no major protocol deviations" (noted in a figure legend only), who were seronegative at baseline, who developed illness with onset at least 14 days after the second injection, and who met the regulatory agencies' requirement of a median follow-up duration of at least two months. This is not an appropriate way of reporting a randomized trial, but there were also data for all the patients, 19 vs. 269 cases, which is a vaccine efficacy of 93.4%.

A secondary end point was severe COVID-19 defined by one of the following criteria: respiratory rate at least 30; pulse at least 125; oxygen saturation at most 93% (or a ratio of the partial pressure of oxygen to the fraction of inspired oxygen below 300 mm Hg); respiratory failure; acute respiratory distress syndrome; evidence of shock (systolic blood pressure less than 90 mm Hg, diastolic blood pressure less than 60 mm Hg, or a need for vasopressors); clinically significant acute renal, hepatic, or neurologic dysfunction; admission to an intensive care unit; or death.

The reporting of adverse events was similarly obscure as in the other *New England Journal of Medicine* article,[94] and a lot was missing or seriously misleading even though these events were described over two pages.

In the main text, adverse events were downplayed, and the reporting was inappropriate. In several cases, adverse events were only reported for the vaccine group, and the grades used for severity were not defined in the article, only in a supplement.

Solicited adverse events at the injection site occurred in 84.2% vs. 19.8% after the first dose and in 88.6% vs. 18.8% after the second dose (number needed to harm only 1.4). The most common harm was pain (88.2% vs. 17.0%). The harms lasted 3 days, on average.

Solicited systemic adverse events occurred in 54.9% vs. 42.2% after the first dose and in 79.4% vs. 36.5% after the second dose. Not only the difference in occurrence (42.9%), but also the severity increased after the second dose, with an increase in grade 3 events from 2.9% to 15.8% in the vaccine group.

There were no data on placebo in the article, but the supplement revealed how bad this really was. The most common harms after the second dose were fever (15.5% vs. 0.3%), headache (58.6% vs. 23.4%), fatigue (65.3% vs. 23.4%), myalgia (58.0% vs. 12.4%), arthralgia (42.8% vs. 10.8%), nausea or vomiting (19.0% vs. 6.4%), and chills (44.2% vs. 5.6%). The systemic harms lasted 3 days, on average.

The grading was explained on page 157 in the supplement: Grade 3 was pretty much the same as a severe adverse event, defined on page 160 as preventing daily activity and requiring intensive therapeutic intervention. Grade 4 was similar to serious adverse events, as it required emergency room visits or hospitalization. These are the data for grades 3 and 4 after the second dose:

	Vaccine N = 14,677	Placebo N = 14,566
Grade 3	2,325 (15.8%)	282 (1.9%)
Grade 4	14 (0.1%)	3 (0.1%)

There could be a printing error in Moderna's table because the percentages for both grade 4 numbers are 0.1. If not, the numbers mean that for every 1,337 patients who are vaccinated, one would need to go to hospital because of a serious systemic harm.

The numbers for grade 3 mean that for every 7 patients vaccinated, one is severely harmed and unable to perform daily activities. The published article did not report on all severe adverse events but only mentioned the unsolicited ones, which were only 234 vs. 202 (1.5% vs. 1.3%), and those unsolicited ones considered treatment-related, only 71 vs. 28 patients (0.5% vs. 0.2%). Using these highly misleading data, numbers needed to harm are 478 and 353, respectively, which are over 50 times higher than the true number of 7 from the supplement. It will escape most readers that the authors only reported on unsolicited harms in the article, as there are 332 words between "unsolicited" and "71." The published article has no information on ALL severe adverse events. This is so misleading that I consider it scientific misconduct, particularly considering that most people only read the abstract, which was even worse: "Moderate, transient reactogenicity after vaccination occurred more frequently" in the vaccine group.

The numbers for serious adverse events were 207 vs. 211. Hypersensitivity reactions were reported in 1.5% vs. 1.1% of the patients; the number needed to harm was 250.

Of the 37 authors on the trial report, 13 (35%) had nothing to declare. Six were employees and held stock in Moderna, 4 were employees of Moderna, 1 had a patent for a COVID-19 vaccine, 4 had grants or fees from other companies, and 9 had grants from the NIH or similar institutions. The paper was tightly controlled by Moderna, which had used three medical writers to, as it was called, assist in drafting the manuscript for submission and for editorial support. These euphemisms can be shortened to: Moderna did it.

Other issues about vaccines

Currently, about 50 vaccines are under clinical evaluation.[95] Results from trials conducted by Pfizer, Moderna, and the Gamaleya National Research Centre (which developed the Russian Sputnik V vaccine) were first "published" in press releases, with claims of over 90% vaccine efficacy.[96]

Science by press release was scorned by the editor of the *Lancet* ("Publishing interim results through a press release is neither good scientific practice nor does it help to build public trust in vaccines") and the editor of *BMJ* ("Science by press release is just one of many flaws in the way new treatments are evaluated"), who pointed to previous fiascos involving remdesivir and Tamiflu.[97] It also leaves stock markets vulnerable to manipulation.

The Gamaleya National Center of Epidemiology and Microbiology in Moscow says about itself that it is the world's leading research institution. Self-praise is not convincing, and the lengthy press release from November 11 about preliminary results obtained with the Sputnik V vaccine is totally devoid of meaningful facts: "Vaccine efficacy amounted to 92% (calculation based on the 20 confirmed COVID-19 cases split between vaccinated individuals and those who received the placebo)."[98] It is impossible to get 92% efficacy if the numbers randomized to vaccine and placebo are about equal: 1 vs. 19 gives 95% and 2 vs. 18 gives 90%. Furthermore, 20 cases are far too little to say much about the efficacy of the vaccine. If we assume the correct numbers are 18 out of 20, the 95% confidence interval for this proportion is 68% to 99%.

Drug firms and authorities have misinformed the public about what the purpose of the vaccine trials is. Moderna called hospital admissions a "key secondary endpoint" in statements to the media, and the NIH stated in a press release that Moderna's trial "seeks to answer if the vaccine can prevent death caused by covid-19."[99] But Moderna's chief medical officer has admitted that the company's trial lacks adequate statistical power to assess these outcomes. None of the vaccine trials have been designed to study them, or to determine if the vaccines can reduce transmission of the virus.[100]

The UK rushed ahead of everyone else and approved the BioNTech-Pfizer vaccine nine days before the FDA did. This caused the Trump administration to call the FDA commissioner to the White House to explain why the United States wasn't the greatest this time.[101]

Noncoronavirus vaccines are also being investigated. A trial has started in the Netherlands where health personnel are vaccinated against tuberculosis because this vaccine also has positive effects against other infections (see Chapter 1). The polio vaccine is another interesting candidate.[102]

Should You Get Vaccinated?

From a public health perspective, it is highly rational to vaccinate broadly based on the knowledge we currently have about the coronavirus vaccines and the devastating consequences of the pandemic.

It is less clear what the individual should do. We should not repeat the mistakes we made with the influenza vaccines, which have never demonstrated an effect on outcomes that really matter. On the other hand, based on the preliminary evidence, the coronavirus vaccines seem to be a lot better than flu shots.

Currently, we know absolutely nothing about long-term harms, and some people have argued that the approvals happened too quickly. Moreover, governments in several countries have given the vaccine manufacturers legal indemnity protecting the companies against being sued by patients for vaccine harms.[103] Thus, the only ones that have acquired 100% immunity are the drug companies.

On this background, it is less surprising that a survey of several countries from December showed that "if there was a COVID-19 vaccine that was proven to be safe and effective," only about two-thirds of the population would take it.[104] In the United States, three-quarters would take it, in Brazil 85%, but in Russia, only 55%.

We do not know for how long the protection lasts, but it could be short-lived. Serial measurements from 452 infected healthcare workers demonstrated that the antibody levels rose to a peak 24 days after the first positive PCR test; had an estimated half-life of only 85 days; and an estimated median time to loss of a positive antibody result of 166 days.[105] The durability is similar to the seasonal coronaviruses, where reinfection can occur within a year, and is much shorter than for those coronaviruses causing SARS and MERS, where most long-term studies have found antibodies up to 1–3 years later. Even though the innate and cellular responses contribute importantly to conferring immunity, these results are worrying.

It seems to me that what we are confronting is similar to a bad influenza. Many mutations of the coronavirus have been described, infectivity and case mortality rates are similar to those of influenza, and acquired immunity after infection is likely to be poor. This suggests that coronavirus vaccines may be ineffective in the long run and that vaccinated people may become infected.

Statistics are absolutely essential but cannot tell the full story. It is also important to listen to patients. A research nurse who participated in Pfizer's trial has described her experiences.[106] After the first injection, her arm was sore. After the second, her arm became much more painful than the first time. By the end of the day, she felt light-headed, chilled, nauseated, and had a splitting headache. She went to bed early but woke up around midnight feeling worse—feverish and chilled, nauseated, dizzy, and hardly able to lift her arm from muscle pain at the injection site. She slept badly, and, in the morning, her temperature was 104.9 °F (40.5 °C). She got scared and reported the harms to the research office. Two days later, her symptoms were gone except for a sore, swollen bump at the injection site. The worst part was that, despite the extensive information she had received, she did not anticipate a reactogenic response. Her gut reaction was: do I have COVID-19? When she texted a few friends about her experience, their response was the same: "Wait, does this mean you have COVID-19? Are you contagious?"

* * *

The American Academy of Family Physicians provides information on the messenger RNA vaccines on its website. It is undated, but a reference shows it was written on December 17 or later.[107]

They write: "An mRNA vaccine . . . can cause mild symptoms in some people (e.g., fatigue, achiness, fever). Based on data from the clinical trials, the most common reactions to the vaccine are pain at the injection site, fatigue, headache, and muscle aches."

This information is seriously misleading, and the dishonesty continues: "By getting vaccinated, you are reducing your risk of disease, hospitalization, severe complications, and even death. Getting vaccinated and reducing the risk of disease also helps prevent the health care system from being further overwhelmed."

Then comes even more wishful thinking and a contradiction: "We do know that seasonal coronaviruses (a source for the common cold) do not induce a robust immune response, which leads to limited immunity to these viruses. It is likely that a vaccine will have a stronger and more lasting immune response, but data are limited and the research is ongoing . . . It is known that natural immunity to the virus wanes over time, so currently, under the EUA [Emergency Use Authorization], individuals who have previously been infected are eligible for receiving the vaccine."

How can the Academy find it likely that the vaccine will have a stronger and more lasting immune response than natural infection with coronaviruses? For vaccines in general, it is the other way around. Natural infection usually provides much better immunity than vaccines.[108]

Our experience with the influenza vaccines (see Chapter 4) suggests that the Academy will not be alone in spreading totally dishonest information to Americans about the benefits and harms of the coronavirus vaccines. This is very sad, as it reduces people's confidence in the advice they receive and therefore increases resistance toward all vaccines.

* * *

The pandemic panic caused the Danish National Board of Health to violate its own guidelines.[109] They plan to vaccinate children against COVID-19 even though the introduction of a vaccination in the childhood vaccination program requires that the disease being vaccinated against must have a certain severity and occurrence and therefore be important to prevent. The severity criterion is the reason why we do not vaccinate children against influenza and chicken pox. COVID-19 is not a serious disease for children, and none of the first 975 Danes who died from COVID-19 were under 30 years of age.

Other criteria that also disqualify the coronavirus vaccines are: "The vaccine must have been tested on larger groups of children to ensure that the vaccine's effect and side effects are known among children" and there must be "sufficient evidence that the benefits of vaccinating against a disease clearly outweigh the risk of harms."

We know that vaccinations with nonlive agents increase the risk of other infections and total mortality (see Chapter 1). There is a risk that by vaccinating children against COVID-19, we will send them on a path where they will have to be vaccinated frequently if the new vaccines do not provide long-term immunity—while they would not have had the same need after natural infection.

For children in low-income countries, UNICEF should prioritize using vaccines with proven benefit to children. Despite the beneficial nonspecific effects of the BCG vaccine against tuberculosis and the measles vaccine, around 30% of the poorest children do not get the BCG vaccine on time or the measles vaccine at all. Both vaccines are associated with almost a halving of the mortality rate among those vaccinated.[110]

* * *

The huge effects touted in press releases, 95% vaccine efficacy, are much smaller in absolute numbers, only 0.84% efficacy.[111] Thus, by getting vaccinated, a person will lower the risk of getting infected in the next two months by a small amount, and we do not know what happens in the ensuing months, only that revaccinations might be needed.

A common argument is that we should vaccinate children to protect the elderly. I find this unethical, particularly because the vaccines cause severe harms and have unknown harms yet to be elucidated.

No one has the right to ask another person about vaccination status. If a doctor is asked by a colleague if she is vaccinated, she can say that she has not had the time yet, or something similar. She should avoid replying, as it is a private matter. We do not want a situation like in former East Germany, where neighbors spied on you and reported to Stasi (the Ministry for State Security, also called the secret police) if they thought you did not comply with what the regime wanted.

* * *

Whether you should get vaccinated or not depends on age, other risk factors, and particularly where you live, as the death risk varies more than 3,000 times between countries.

If you live in Taiwan, I cannot see any good reason for getting vaccinated. But let us assume you live in Denmark and are between 50 and 59 years old. In 2020, 36 people in this age group died from COVID-19,[112] which is 1.1% of all deaths.[113] Thus, your risk of dying of COVID-19 is only about 1% of your total risk of dying.

Most of the other causes of death are beyond our control, but some are not. If you smoke, for example, it is more important to stop smoking than to get vaccinated. For all age groups, the table looks like this:

Age group	Deaths	Corona Deaths	Risk
0-39	983	3	0.3%
40-49	1,046	1	0.1%
50-59	3,270	36	1.1%
60-69	7,295	115	1.6%
70-79	14,271	347	2.4%
80+	28,367	796	2.7%
Total	55,232	1,298	2.3%

A recent paper using data from 45 countries found that, from age 30, there is a log-linear increase in COVID-19 mortality by age.[114] This is scary news for old people, but it is misleading, as it does not take into account that competing death risks increase with age.

By far most people who die from COVID-19 have serious comorbidity. If you don't have that, your relative risk of dying from COVID-19 will be much lower than shown in the table. If you mix little with crowds, your risk will also be much lower. You might also consider that even after a year with COVID-19, the Danish death toll (all ages) is still at the same level as our annual deaths from influenza and that the median age at death is over 80 (in the United States, it is around 80).[115] Thus, if you don't get flu shots, then why should you get a coronavirus vaccine?

People in leading positions in Denmark, e.g., the director of the drug agency, have come forward on TV and declared that they will get vaccinated. Celebrity announcements have a huge influence on people. I therefore provide a little balance by declaring that I shall not get a coronavirus vaccine, at least not now. My age is at the upper end of the table, but I am in good shape, with no risk factors. Some people will call me irresponsible, but derogatory adjectives help no one, and my decision is based on the facts.

Pandemrix, an influenza vaccine, caused narcolepsy (see Chapter 4). Even though the risk is presumably very small, I would never forgive myself if I became seriously and irreversibly harmed by a coronavirus vaccine. The situation is totally different for the measles vaccine, which we know much more about and which I believe we should all take in solidarity with other people in order to obtain herd immunity.

In the corona vaccine trials, 7 vs. 1 patients developed Bell's palsy, which is a one-sided facial paralysis with a good prognosis. This does not worry me, and it could easily be a chance finding. Unfortunately, vaccine deniers are spreading a lot of worries about people who have died after a coronavirus vaccine, which is only expected given the average age people have. As just noted, my expectation is that the vaccines will lower mortality dramatically. But I shall wait and see what happens when millions of people have been vaccinated before I possibly change my mind.

Greed, Corruption, and Unethical and Unlawful Interventions

It is during humanitarian crises that we can see clearly if we have good leaders and if people's moral compasses are intact.

Early on, commercial vendors took advantage of the crisis. Supplies could take months to deliver, market manipulation was widespread, and stocks were often sold to the highest bidder. Prices of gowns doubled, prices of respirators more than tripled, and prices of face masks increased sixfold.[116] The panic caused the public to purchase so many face masks that it caused a shortage at hospitals.

There was also corruption. Little is known about the interests of the doctors and scientists on whose advice our governments rely to manage the pandemic.[117] Corporate interests are always granted access to government decision makers, whereas the public is kept in the dark. When the *BMJ* sought further information, the information was denied, or requests were unanswered.

BMJ's executive editor wrote a scathing editorial in November explaining how COVID-19 has unleashed state corruption on a grand scale where science is being suppressed by politicians for political and financial gain, and also where industry, scientists, and health experts have contributed to the opportunistic embezzlement.[118]

The membership, research, and deliberations of the UK Scientific Advisory Group for Emergencies (SAGE) were initially secret until a press leak forced transparency. The leak revealed inappropriate involvement of government advisers in SAGE, while exposing underrepresentation from public health, clinical care, women, and ethnic minorities who have been hit the most by the pandemic.

The publication of a Public Health England report on COVID-19 and inequalities was delayed by England's Department of Health. Following a public outcry, a section on ethnic minorities, which was initially withheld, was published as part of a follow-up report. But authors from Public Health England were instructed not to talk to the media. A UK government scientist who had published a research paper was also blocked by the government from speaking to media because of a "difficult political landscape."

The prime minister introduced mass screening based on an antibody test that, in real world tests, falls well short of performance claims made by its manufacturers. Researchers from Public Health England and collaborating institutions pushed to publish their study findings on the poor performance before the government committed to buying a million of these tests but were blocked by the health department and the prime minister's office. Subsequently, Public Health England unsuccessfully attempted to block the *BMJ*'s press release about the research paper.

Even though expertise is possible without competing interests, the United Kingdom's pandemic response relies heavily on scientists and other government appointees with worrying competing interests, including shareholdings in companies that manufacture COVID-19 diagnostic tests, treatments, and vaccines. Government appointees are able to ignore or cherry-pick science and indulge in anti-competitive practices that favor their own products and those of friends and associates.

The UK government also showed little concern that advisers to the coronavirus Vaccine Taskforce have financial interests in pharmaceutical companies receiving government contracts.[119]

The scope for corruption is gigantic. In July, the government signed a coronavirus vaccine deal for an undisclosed sum with GlaxoSmithKline, securing 60 million doses of an untested treatment that was still being developed. The government's chief scientific adviser is Sir Patrick Vallance, who was president of Research and Development at GlaxoSmithKline from 2012 to 2018 and owned shares in the company worth £600,000. Astonishingly, when confronted with this, the minister of health denied that there was a conflict of interest, and when asked when he learned about it, he said, "Well, I didn't know about it until I read it in the newspapers."[120]

Another nobleman, but not a noble man, Sir John Bell, had £773,000 worth of shares in Roche, which had sold the government £13.5m of antibody tests in May. Following the deal, Bell appeared on Channel 4 News and Radio 4's *Today*, calling the tests a major step forward. Yet Public Health England found the tests unreliable.

When the *BMJ* approached Bell's employer, Oxford University, to ask for documents that confirmed that he had disclosed his financial interests, the request was denied: "Professor Sir John Bell has always declared his financial interests and board membership at Roche, in accordance with the university's conflict of interest policy for all staff."

This is a European country. It is not Russia, although it looks like it. Transparency is the vaccine against corruption, but this vaccine is much underused, as it leads to economic losses for powerful people.

When Pfizer announced that its vaccine was highly effective, global stocks soared and Pfizer's chief executive, Albert Bourla, sold US$5.6 million of stock at a whisker from the company's all-time high.[121] If Bourla had sold his stock a day before the press release, he would have earned US$0.8 million less.

Moderna's chief executive, Stéphane Bancel, sold a whopping US$49.8 million of shares in the company.

No wonder that vaccines and other drugs are so expensive. But the prices of the vaccines were kept secret by the European Commission with the lame excuse that it would weaken the European Union's position in future negotiations.[122] The Commission has adopted this bullshit argument directly from the drug industry that prefers that everything be top secret. If it weren't, there would be much less corruption.

A Belgian minister tweeted the prices as part of a debate about government expenses, but her Tweet was removed with lightning speed. Pfizer was first to criticize her, but thanks to her courage, we know what the prices were for one dose of the vaccines:[123]

Oxford-AstraZeneca	1.78 €
Johnson & Johnson	7.00 €
Sanofi-GlaxoSmithKline	7.56 €
Curevac	10.00 €
BioNTech-Pfizer	12.00 €
NIH-Moderna	14.75 €

Mandatory flu shots
I have already argued why mandatory vaccinations are a bad idea (see Chapter 3). It becomes particularly bad when authorities make it mandatory to become vaccinated against influenza to lower the burden on

overstretched hospital departments. This is both unethical and unscientific. Flu shots do not reduce hospital admissions or days off work (see Chapter 4).

On her last day of work, on July 31, University of California President Janet Napolitano issued an executive order mandating flu shots for all students, faculty, and employees (around 510,000) as a condition of continued employment and continued school enrollment for students. The justification was to mitigate a possible future shortage of hospital beds, if there was a second wave of COVID-19 and if there was a big seasonal flu outbreak.

This was a tremendous human rights violation.[124] In California, and in the rest of America, too, only one-third of adults get an influenza vaccination.[125] In a declaration in support of plaintiffs' motion for a preliminary injunction to the superior court, I explained that, among other things, Napolitano in her executive order quoted the literature selectively to such an extent that I considered it scientific misconduct according to the definition used by the US Office of Research Integrity.

A problem with judges is that they often focus too little on the evidence and too much on authority, which also happened here. Our motion was denied even though the other side only provided opinions and personal experiences while we provided solid scientific arguments.

The judge made credibility determinations. The other side had specialists in infectious diseases whose views were in line with the CDC's strong recommendations that everyone should get a flu shot. It would take a brave judge to go against prevailing medical and public health opinion during a pandemic. The judge also let his private views play a role. He said he would be afraid of sitting next to someone who wasn't flu-vaccinated and made a ridiculous analogy to drunk driving.

We would expect flu shots to increase the risk of serious COVID-19 (see Chapter 1), which was confirmed in a large observational study of people aged 65 and above from 39 countries.[126] COVID-19 deaths per million and the case fatality rate were both associated with the influenza vaccination rate (p < 0.001). The degree of lockdown and the degree of requirement for mask use in public were not associated with mortality rates.

A study performed in two US states compared 4,138 patients who received unadjuvanted influenza vaccination in the fall of 2019 or winter of 2020 with 9,082 who had never received influenza vaccination.[127] The report is very brief, only 750 words. It showed that vaccinated individuals were less likely to test positive for coronavirus. However, among those who tested positive, influenza vaccination increased the risk of hospitalization, admission to the intensive care unit, and death. There were huge differences between vaccinated and unvaccinated people, e.g., the average ages were 62 and 49, respectively, and the vaccinated people had more coexisting conditions. In adjusted analyses, the differences in testing positive for coronavirus and bad outcomes were gone.

Both studies should be interpreted cautiously, as those vaccinated are not comparable to those not vaccinated, but they suggest that previous influenza vaccination might make matters worse.

Human challenge trials

To accelerate the development of vaccines, "human challenge trials" are underway in the United Kingdom with government support of £33.6 million where volunteers will be deliberately infected with the coronavirus in a "secure quarantine facility."[128] The researchers did not want to comment publicly ahead of the launch. I cannot understand why there has not been a public outcry. How could anyone—after the Nuremberg trials and the Declaration of Helsinki—get to the point of accepting to expose volunteers to a virus that has killed 3 million people worldwide?

People in favor of such trials have argued that the risk of dying for young volunteers is similar to the risk of live kidney donation, and Dominic Wilkinson, professor of medical ethics at Oxford University, stated that "When we are facing an unprecedented global threat from COVID, it is an ethical imperative to carry out well-controlled challenge studies to help develop a vaccine and then to identify the best vaccines."[129]

These arguments are invalid. We are not allowed to expose people to unacceptable risks in order to benefit others, which is what the Nazis did in the concentration camps. It is also wrong to call this an ethical imperative. Finally, when people donate a kidney, it is usually because they wish to help a suffering, concrete relative.

The trialists consider it essential to have a "rescue remedy" on hand to prevent serious illness in participants, and a trial in London will initially use remdesivir. However, as we have seen, this drug does not work.

Volunteers who take part in influenza challenge studies receive up to £3,750 compensation. The payment for the COVID-19 trials is likely to be higher because the isolation will last longer—potentially as long as a month.

These trials are hugely immoral. And who will the volunteers be? Likely poorer than average. I am appalled that this can happen.

The killing of 17 million mink in Denmark

After a mutation was found in Danish mink, which laboratory studies at the State Serum Institute had shown would make a vaccine less effective, Prime Minister Mette Frederiksen ordered all Danish mink exterminated immediately.[130] This order was illegal, and one of the mass graves was also illegal, as it was much too close to a lake. Other mass graves posed a pollution risk to the drinking water supply. In addition, the graves were too shallow, and the decomposing bodies of the mink soon resurfaced as what the media dubbed "zombie mink." Many of the mink will likely get exhumed and burnt.

Denmark was the largest producer of pelts in the world, and we had three times as many mink as people. Coronavirus has also been found in mink on farms in the United States, Spain, and the Netherlands, and Spain and the Netherlands have carried out partial culls. In the Netherlands, five mutant mink strains of coronavirus did not spread beyond mink farmworkers, and the mutant in Danish mink had likely died out two months before the mass killing was ordered.

Kåre Mølbak, the outgoing head of the State Serum Institute, had warned at an internal meeting with the government that the mink farms could become a new Wuhan, but when journalists later found this out and asked for a comment, he refused.

The prime minister, for a minority government, acted dictatorially without involving the Parliament, which was another huge mistake and unlike the consensus-seeking approach that dominates Danish politics.

A week after the mass killings, Danish experts had read a report the State Serum Institute had issued about the danger the new mutant posed, and they all concluded that it was not dangerous.[131] There was no reason to expect that the vaccines would not work. The mutant was less sensitive toward the antibodies, but it was still sensitive.

In the middle of this huge scandal, I was interviewed in the news and I asked what we should do if we encountered a pandemic of swine flu and a mutation arose in Danish pigs. Should we then also kill all our 25 million pigs? We cannot go on like this. The Danish prime minister killed a whole profession overnight for no good reason.

The nanny state

By the end of 2020, elderly people living in a nursing home in Denmark were forced to choose just one family member to visit them.[132] The health minister's argument was that we needed to take extra good care of the residents because a third of all COVID-19 deaths have occurred in nursing homes. With this type of argument, we could also ban all young men from driving because most deaths in traffic happen among young men.

The minister's unsolicited guardianship of persons who are legally competent and entitled to autonomy cannot be defended. In principle, paternalism is a good thing because it is about taking care of the interests of others, but this is unsolicited paternalism, where the elderly did not give permission for others to intervene on their behalf (see Chapter 3).

Many old people have very little time left to live, which they are well aware of, and they would rather run a slightly increased risk of becoming infected than not seeing and hugging their loved ones, but the minister did not allow them this.

It is a dangerous path for our democracies when the state knows best and violates human rights. History has shown that leaders who assure us that the situation is so grave that we must give up our freedom or ethical principles, or both, to gain security against an external or internal danger usually end up giving us neither freedom nor security, but absolute power to themselves.

It went so far that Head of Cabinet Per Okkels wrote to Director of the National Board of Health Søren Brostrøm that he should abandon his professionalism for political reasons.[133] This is also dangerous. If truth doesn't matter, and those who hold the power can lie as they please, creating a false reality, we pave the way for the introduction of a dictatorship. We have seen far too many of these in Europe in the last 100 years. Think of Russia, Belarus, Portugal, Spain, Germany, Italy, Albania, Romania, Bulgaria, Hungary, Poland, Czechoslovakia, East Germany, and Greece, and the millions of killings and unimaginable sufferings the dictatorships brought with them. We even have them today, just outside the European Union, and new ones are on their way, in Poland and Hungary.

The Danish government sent both the police and military to North Jutland to scare the lives out of the mink farmers, even though the extermination order was illegal. This is what we see when a country moves from being a democracy to becoming a dictatorship. It worries me.

Testing Mania

For the most of 2020, every time we turned on the news, it was corona, corona, corona. We have never before seen nonstop media coverage with every talking head, opinion columnist, or self-appointed amateur expert weighing in on how it is going. In Denmark, our lives were pestered by daily counts of new cases, admissions, and deaths, as well as endless press conferences with the prime minister, the minister of health, and the heads of the Board of Health, the Serum Institute, and the police, who were all constantly worried and asked for further sacrifices.

It was like a new worldwide religion, something that was supposed to unite us, as if eternal life lay ahead if only we did not die from COVID-19.

"Test, test, test," said WHO's director general on TV. But whom and how often? Testing is essential for contact tracing, but testing most of the population repeatedly is irrational. The Danish government announced in December that they had made it possible to test over 200,000 Danes per day. This means that the whole population can be tested every month, at a price of 1.4 billion Euros a year, or far more if people go to private test centers.

This is totally crazy. The mass testing is also hugely expensive in terms of human suffering.[134] The PCR tests were never designed to be used across entire populations with no symptoms, which yields far too many false positives; they are a tool to help with diagnosis. Dr. Tom Jefferson has written extensively about the pandemic and receives many emails from desperate people who test positive long after any possible infection, who flip-flop between positive and negative tests, or who cannot visit their loves ones in care homes because they test positive week after week. "These individuals are trapped, prisoners of the testing regime."[135]

These tests are the standard PCR tests. Even though the duration of viable virus is only up to 8 days, the virus can be detected by PCR up to 83 days after the infection.[136]

A UK study performed over two days in April showed that, of 545 asymptomatic healthcare workers who all agreed to be tested, viral carriage was detected by PCR in 2.4% and antibodies in 24.4%.[137] This is a huge prevalence rate of infection, compared to the general population.

The PCR test used in this study had 100% sensitivity and 97.8% specificity. This is a highly accurate test if used when infection is suspected. But it performs poorly when used as a screening test. If we assume that out of 1,000 people going to a test center, 10 are infected and 990 are not (a disease prevalence of 1%), we may construct this table:

	Infected	Healthy
Test +	10	22
Test -	0	968

Thus, only 31% (10 of 32) of the people who test positive with a swab and a PCR test are infected, whereas the other 69% are not. If the percentage of positive tests is 0.5%, which it currently is in Denmark, it is only 19% of those who test positive who are infected.

As Jefferson wrote: "We must bring this indiscriminate regime of mass tests to a halt, concentrating instead on those who have good reason to believe they have the virus."[138]

Should We Do Everything Possible in Virus Pandemics?

An often-heard argument in favor of draconian measures is that we should do our utmost to limit the number of deaths, at any cost, as we should not set a price on a human life. This was the interviewer's main argument when I was interviewed on Sky News in April. He considered it cynical to set a price on a human life. But we already do this. There is an economic and a societal limit as to what we can do. We could avoid virtually all traffic deaths if we lowered the speed limit for all vehicles to walking speed.

If we had no limits, we could use the entire gross national product on helping people survive from all sorts of diseases.

If we focused on things other than containing the current pandemic, we could avoid many more deaths. Millions of people die every year from malaria, tuberculosis, diarrhea, and many other infections, and the number of healthy life years lost is formidable, as, in contrast to COVID-19, many people die young.

If we had drug regulators who didn't see themselves as service personnel for the drug industry but as guardians of public health, we could help millions survive every year, as most of those killed by prescription drugs didn't need them.[139] It cannot be repeated too often that medications are the third-leading cause of death after heart disease and cancer.

If we made tobacco illegal or increased the tax on cigarettes substantially, we could help other millions survive. Instead of daily numbers of deaths caused by corona, I would prefer to see daily numbers of tobacco deaths and authorities who constantly worried about this and held press conferences. On average, smokers lose 10 years of their life, many die relatively young, and many suffer horribly for several years before they die.

We need to get away from the misleading notion that we save lives. We can only extend lives, and the lives we extend are already aged. Economic estimates have shown that the price we pay to extend lives during the coronavirus pandemic exceeds vastly anything we have ever accepted before. In

March, the US Government had set aside $2 trillion to deal with the pandemic, and in the United Kingdom, it was over £350 billion, almost three times the annual budget for the entire National Health Service.[140]

The UK National Institute for Health and Care Excellence (NICE) will recommend funding medical interventions if they cost less than £30,000 per quality-adjusted life year (QALY). If 20,000 deaths are prevented, the cost per QALY is around £7 million. The government estimated 250,000 as the upper limit of deaths if nothing was done to prevent spread, and if all these deaths were prevented—which is totally unrealistic, of course—the cost per QALY is around £400,000.[141]

A quick look at Danish figures shows a much worse outcome than the overoptimistic UK guesswork. In early October, the cost for Denmark was estimated at 207 billion Danish crowns.[142] In December, the difference in COVID-19 deaths between Sweden and Denmark was 613 per million inhabitants, which translates to 3,555 avoided deaths in Denmark at a rough cost of 8 million Euros per person aged 82 on average who did not die from COVID-19. This is somewhat exaggerated, as Sweden has also had costs related to the pandemic, but it tells us that our priorities are wrong and are the result of fear, political expediency, greed, and corruption. As Professor Thorkild IA Sørensen put it, an 82-year-old could say: "OK, I made it this time but are you willing to pay the same amount to save me from dying from my next disease?"

We also need to think of the opportunity cost, which is the loss of other alternatives when one alternative is chosen. Some elderly people with lack of support die of dehydration and starvation. Many people with other diseases do not get the attention and treatment they need, which has increased suffering and deaths substantially. In the United States, many emergency visits have disappeared, and a huge number of patients with heart attacks and ischemic strokes have not turned up at hospitals, likely because they are afraid of getting infected with coronavirus.[143] Since the chance of survival for both conditions is closely related to how fast you get treated with thrombolytics, the death toll is considerable. In America, about 800,000 die every year from heart disease or stroke.[144]

At the other end of the age spectrum, it is much worse. It has been estimated that lockdowns, lack of staff, and fear of getting infected have increased maternal and child mortality in low-income and middle-income countries so much that hundreds of thousands or perhaps even millions of lives have already been lost.[145] Here, we are not talking about gaining a few years of life at the upper end of the life spectrum, but about loss of lives right from life's beginning, childbirth, and the deaths of tens of thousands of young mothers.

The lockdowns also kill through poverty. In October, the World Bank estimated that the coronavirus pandemic had caused an increase of about 100 million people living in extreme poverty.[146] After India introduced a lockdown, migrant laborers feared that hunger would kill them before the coronavirus did.[147]

Thus, my superficial estimate of a cost of 8 million Euros per person aged 82 whose life is extended thanks to our draconian measures against coronavirus is likely far too optimistic. Looking at the whole world, I find it likely that we have lost many more life years than we have gained.

There has not been much debate about the impact of the economic damage, but it can be immense. The breakdown of the Soviet Union caused economic and social chaos, and in men, life expectancy fell by almost seven years, over a 2–3-year period.[148]

In July, a UK government report estimated that the lockdown could cost 200,000 lives.[149] By October, the United States had an estimated 225,000 excess deaths, and the societal disruption was massive.[150] When businesses go bankrupt, millions lose their jobs and feelings of despair increase and mental health deteriorates. Isolating people in their homes and asking them to work from home increase domestic violence.

A CDC survey from June found that 41% of adults reported at least one adverse mental or behavioral health condition, including depression, anxiety, posttraumatic stress, and substance abuse, with rates that were 3 to 4 times the rates one year earlier, and a stunning 11% of the respondents reported seriously considering suicide in the prior month.

The psychiatrists' response to this challenge was devastating.[151] They suggested screening for mental disorders, which is an exceedingly bad idea,[152] and, even worse, that treatment of those at greatest risk by mental health professionals should involve "judicious use of psychiatric medications." There is no such thing as a "judicious use of psychiatric medications" in people at risk of suicide. Depression pills increase suicides, both in children and adults.[153] People at risk of suicide should receive psychotherapy, which has been shown to halve the risk of a new suicide attempt in those who have already tried.[154] Usage of depression pills went up 19% in the United States compared to a year earlier,[155] which is a disaster.

Scientific, Civil, and Uncensored Debates Are Needed

Many people prefer false certainty to honest uncertainty when they become panic-stricken. This is unhealthy. Hardened positions, which leave little room for uncertainty, nuance, and enlightened debate, undermine public trust as various assertions prove wrong,[156] and it also leads to censorship.

We have not had frank and trustful public discussions about what we should do and not do. Our politicians have consulted with whomever they preferred and have introduced measures that have been immensely harmful to our societies in a shroud of secrecy, where the citizens were kept in the dark even when journalists asked what the scientific basis was for the draconian measures, as people refused to reply.

It should be punishable by law when civil servants or politicians who work for taxpayers' money decline to comment in order to protect themselves, forgetting they are paid to take care of the taxpayers' interests.

The things that give order, perspective, and predictability to our lives have been dismantled with little objection and often without warning. Even though numbers of infected people do not suddenly jump upward, our governments have often announced that from the very next day, all arrangements involving more than a few persons would need to be canceled, which has caused havoc and economic ruin for many people.

The two main ways to respond to a pandemic like COVID-19 were described in the Great Barrington Declaration on October 4[157] and the John Snow Memorandum on October 14.[158]

The Great Barrington Declaration takes up only 514 words, and there are no references. I did not find anything in it to be factually wrong.

It emphasizes the devastating effects of lockdowns on short- and long-term public health, with the underprivileged disproportionately harmed. Arguing that for children, COVID-19 is less dangerous than influenza, it suggests that those at minimal risk of death should live their lives normally to build up immunity to the virus through natural infection and to establish herd immunity in the society.

It recommends an approach called Focused Protection, which is about protecting the vulnerable. Nursing homes should use staff with acquired immunity and perform frequent PCR testing of other staff and all visitors. Retired people living at home should have groceries and other essentials delivered to their home and should meet family members outside when possible.

Staying home when sick should be practiced by everyone; schools, universities, sports facilities, restaurants, cultural activities, and other businesses should be open. Young low-risk adults should work normally, rather than from home.

The John Snow Memorandum was published in the *Lancet*. It is 945 words, with 8 references. It is seriously manipulative. There are factual inaccuracies, and several references are to highly unreliable science. The authors claim that SARS-CoV-2 has high infectivity, and that the infection fatality rate of COVID-19 is severalfold higher than that of seasonal influenza. Both claims are wrong, and the two references they use are to studies that have used modeling, which is highly bias-prone.

They also claim that transmission of the virus can be mitigated through the use of face masks, with no reference, even though this is also wrong.

They write that "the proportion of vulnerable people constitute as much as 30% of the population in some regions." This is fearmongering and cherry-picking from yet another modeling study whose authors defined increased risk of severe disease as one of the conditions listed in current guidelines."[159] With such a broad definition, it is easy to scare people. However, they also estimated that only 4% of the global population would require hospital admission if infected, which is rather similar to influenza.

These two declarations did not elicit enlightened debates, but acrimonious exchanges of views on social media and email lists dominated by strong emotions devoid of facts. The vitriolic attacks have almost exclusively been directed against those supporting the ideas in the Great Barrington Declaration.

* * *

Academic bullying and ad hominem attacks in relation to discussions about how we should handle the pandemic have created groupthink, have caused serious reputational harm, and have led some scientists to self-censor and avoid publishing data that could potentially reduce death rates.[160] Some researchers have even refused to talk to journalists anonymously.

Professor John Ioannidis from Stanford University, the world's most cited medical researcher, became the subject of one of the worst witch hunts in recent medical history, described by journalists Jeanne Lenzer and Shannon Brownlee in *Scientific American*.[161] In March, Ioannidis expressed concerns that we lacked data on the benefits and harms of lockdowns and other draconian responses to the outbreak. He estimated that deaths in the United States from COVID-19 could potentially be as low as 10,000 or they could approach levels not seen since the flu pandemic in 1918.[162] He pleaded for better science in order to make informed decisions.

Fellow researchers latched on to his low figure, accusing him of horrible science and of missing the point by calling for more data when coffins of victims were accumulating. Detractors even falsely accused him of recommending that the nation should do nothing in response to the virus.

When Ioannidis was interviewed a week later, he said that "We're falling into a trap of sensationalism" and that "We have gone into a complete panic state."[163] The video was viewed more than a half-million times before YouTube took it down, saying the interview violated its policies on COVID-19 misinformation. I have not seen the video, but it is correct that the whole world panicked and that a lot of sensational claims were circulated, often with wild exaggerations about how dangerous the virus was.

Obscene and defamatory emails were sent to Ioannidis and his administrators and colleagues at Stanford.[164] Numerous erroneous claims were advanced in the press, including the charge that he had a financial conflict of interest related to a study he coauthored. He was fiercely attacked when he published a study to determine the percentage of people in Santa Clara County infected with COVID-19.[165] Critics accused him of being a right-wing Trump supporter after he had appeared on a number of Fox News shows and had written to Trump of his concerns about the lack of evidence regarding the efficacy of lockdowns.

Ioannidis is my friend, and he supported me when I was kicked out of Cochrane for telling people what I had observed, just like Ioannidis does (see next chapter). If he had consulted me, I would strongly have discouraged him from writing to Trump and from appearing on Trump's favorite news channel, which is a mastermind in fake news and horrendous lies.

Ioannidis came under more fire when he published an analysis showing that the infection fatality rate of COVID-19 was far lower than initially reported.[166] It did not matter that he was right again, or that the CDC later published similarly low rates, or that WHO published a systematic review by Ioannidis, which confirmed his initial findings.[167]

Scientific American committed editorial misconduct.[168] The editors uploaded "corrections" on the journal's homepage, several of which were errors committed by themselves, and others were not true or irrelevant. They violated the first rule of journalistic integrity by publishing accusations without inquiring of the accused. Lenzer and Brownlee tried to correct the false "corrections," but the editors denied them also this opportunity. The inappropriate "corrections" triggered an outpouring of hate mail and false claims about Ioannidis and the integrity of Lenzer and Brownlee as journalists.

It was so bad that Jeffrey S. Flier, former dean at Harvard Medical School, wrote to the editors asking them to take proper action: By "printing a lengthy correction to their article, while refusing to permit them the opportunity to address the inaccuracies therein, *Scientific American* has needlessly besmirched the reputations of two distinguished and accomplished journalists who deserve a great deal of credit for their work over the years, including efforts to expose problematic issues in biomedical science."[169]

Flier also noted that "By bowing to the mob that has been attacking Ioannidis with false accusations that distort the totality of his work, *Scientific American* has lent support to behaviors that violate the norms of ethical scientific conduct . . . Your statement that Lenzer and Brownlee failed to disclose . . . prior co-authorships implied they were material events the authors were seeking to hide. Unlike many financial relationships, co-authorships are public knowledge—as a quick search of PubMed will show. The norms of scientific publishing would not consider these to be reportable COIs [conflicts of interest]." This was about the fact that Lenzer and Brownlee had once coauthored pieces with Ioannidis and another researcher.

Since I write about Lenzer and Brownlee, I'd better declare that I have met with both of them and appreciate them just as much as Flier does.

Misconduct should always be exposed. Lenzer has published Flier's letter and her and Brownlee's corrections on her website,[170] and I have given a short account of the affair on the website of my Institute for Scientific Freedom.[171]

* * *

The highly anticipated results of the only randomized trial of mask wearing against COVID-19 infection was rejected by *New England Journal of Medicine*, *JAMA*, and the *Lancet*[172] and went unpublished for five months. When the paper appeared in *Annals of Internal Medicine*, an accompanying editorial asked: "With fierce resistance to mask recommendations by leaders and the public in some locales, is it irresponsible for *Annals* to publish these results, which could easily be misused by those opposed to mask recommendations?"[173]

Of course not. Censorship and bullying are what is irresponsible. After the trial was published, Carl Heneghan, professor of evidence-based medicine at the University of Oxford, wrote that "the evidence shows that wearing masks in the community does not significantly reduce the rates of infection."[174] His statement was absolutely correct, but Sonia Sodha, who undersigned herself as "chief leader writer at the *Observer* and a *Guardian* and *Observer* columnist," wrote a piece in *The Guardian* with this head-line: "We need scientists to quiz Covid consensus, not act as agents of disinformation."

Sodha's disinformation continued: "Attacking the science around masks is just one tactic that the anti-science lobby uses to undermine confidence in public health advice. When Facebook rightly classified Heneghan's piece as false information, rather than engage with the substance of the critique, he took to social media to tweet: 'What has happened to academic freedom and freedom of speech?', a message shared widely by prominent mask sceptics. Academic freedom does not imply freedom to spread disinformation."[175]

Which was exactly what Sodha did. Being short of rational arguments, she also used the familiar tactic of name calling. Heneghan's correct inter-pretation of the science does not make him "anti-science" or a "prominent mask sceptic."

Heneghan is also a friend of mine, but this declaration won't keep agents of disinformation off my back. They do not respect the rules the rest of us abide by.

In Sweden, doctors have been bullied and their jobs threatened for speaking out against the country's open approach.[176] A French postdoc-toral fellow in Sweden received multiple death threats after he made com-ments about Didier Raoult, the French researcher who falsely claimed that hydroxychloroquine was effective for the treatment of COVID-19.

The censorship is everywhere. Stefan Baral, an epidemiologist at Johns Hopkins Center for Global Health, reports that a letter he wrote about the potential harms of population-wide lockdowns was rejected by more than 10 scientific journals and 6 newspapers in April, sometimes with the pre-tense that there was nothing useful in it. It was the first time in his career that he could not get a piece placed anywhere.

* * *

Politicization of science was enthusiastically deployed by some of history's worst autocrats and dictators, and it is now regrettably commonplace in democracies.[177] The medical-political complex tends toward suppression of science to aggrandize and enrich those in power. And, as the powerful become more successful, richer, and further intoxicated with power, the inconvenient truths of science are further suppressed.

When good science is suppressed, people die. And when derogatory labels are used, rational conversation dies. According to Merriam-Webster, which calls itself "America's most useful and respected dictionary," UNESCO seems to be an anti-vaxxer agency because it opposes treatment without informed consent. An anti-vaxxer is "a person who opposes vaccination or laws that mandate vaccination."

To ask for a little freedom is almost like being an enemy of the state, it seems. We are moving in the wrong direction.

What Should We Do in the Future?

Knowledge accumulates rapidly, and the Centre for Evidence-Based Medicine in Oxford has a helpful website with analyses and reviews that are regularly updated.[178]

As the COVID-19 pandemic has so clearly illustrated, concern and fear may drive events much more than the disease itself.[179] In 2005, WHO stated that an estimated 2 to 7.4 million people would die from the avian flu, which WHO even called "a relatively conservative estimate."[180] Four years later, the UK government predicted that 65,000 citizens might die during the 2009 swine flu pandemic, but fewer than 500 died.[181]

With such dire predictions, it is reasonable to ask why the draconian measures we have applied now were not applied before. I don't know the answer. But once a country has taken drastic measures, such as lockdowns and border closings, other countries are accused of being irresponsible if they don't take the same actions—even though their effect is unproven. Politicians will not get in trouble for measures that are too draconian, only if it can be argued that they did too little.

Already in March, Ioannidis predicted that total lockdowns might need to continue for very long to have the desired effect.[182] An additional problem is that it is always winter somewhere. We cannot lock down the whole world more or less permanently, and people are fed up with all the restrictions on their daily lives. No one ever asked the whole world to make extraordinary efforts to reduce the number of deaths from influenza. And even so-called mild or common cold-type coronaviruses can have case fatality rates as high as 8% when they infect elderly people in nursing homes.[183]

In the next pandemic, scientists should be involved right from the start, and everything politicians would like to do should be tested in randomized trials, if we don't know if it causes more good than harm. Closure of institutions, restaurants, and sports facilities, size of permitted gatherings, distance between people, mass killing of domestic animals, almost everything can be tested in trials, but we tested virtually nothing during the COVID-19 pandemic and therefore learned very little.

We should act like Taiwan, with aggressive early contact tracing, testing of suspected or possible cases, and isolation outside the home. We should avoid drastic lockdowns but live normally as much as possible while we try to protect the most vulnerable. I believe we have reliable evidence that the draconian COVID-19 lockdowns have caused more harm than good. A comparison of regions in 10 countries showed no additional effect of major lockdowns compared to minor ones.[184] It seems we are destroying our societies and economies for no good reason.

I do not consider wearing face masks as living normally. Many people hate them, and randomized trials did not find they worked. They could be tested in bigger trials, but it is wrong to mandate them given the evidence we currently have.

We have acquired many deadly virus infections from animals, e.g., coronavirus, swine flu, bird flu, AIDS, ebola, rabies, and yellow fever. It would be preferable to close the open animal markets in Southeast Asia where hygiene is nonexistent.

* * *

America is a special case. In contrast to other Western nations, the United States has a weak public health infrastructure, and its response to the pandemic has been decentralized and inconsistent.

A US commentator wrote that the coronavirus didn't break America, it revealed what was already broken: "Years of attacking government, squeezing it dry and draining its morale, inflict a heavy cost that the public has to pay in lives. All the programs defunded, stockpiles depleted, and plans scrapped meant that we had become a second-rate nation."[185]

America has the most ineffective healthcare system in the developed world. The privatized system means that it is doubly as expensive as healthcare systems in Europe, measured as the fraction of the gross national product spent on it, and yet, the healthy life expectancy is considerably worse.[186] The health disadvantage of Americans is not only because of extreme income inequalities and widespread poverty. It is also seen among those with health insurance, a college education, higher incomes, and healthy behaviors,[187] likely because rich Americans tend to be overdiagnosed, overtreated, and overweight. All patients in Moderna's vaccine trial were Americans, and they were about 20 kg overweight on average.[188]

A 2008 report from the Commonwealth Fund found that the United States ranked last among 19 industrialized countries across a range of measures of healthcare.[189] The report estimated that if the country attained the same performance indicators achieved in other industrialized countries, at least 100,000 lives and at least $100 billion could be saved every year.

But truth-telling has become difficult. The political propaganda and lies have made nearly half of all Americans believe that the United States has the best healthcare in the world, albeit with a clear political divide, 68% of Republicans and 32% of Democrats.[190]

When presidential candidates come along who have no plans of increasing the immense wealth gap by tax cuts but care about racial discrimination and the poor and want to ensure that all can get the healthcare they need, monstrous lies are spread about them on Fox News and by ultraconservative commentators like Rush Limbaugh. Former President Barack Obama describes this eloquently in his heartbreaking memoir.[191]

When Democrats try to improve healthcare, Republicans and their supporters cry "socialized medicine," which is used as a derogatory term, even though it only means healthcare for all, ensured through public financing. No one with his or her heart in the right place can be against this, particularly not in such a rich country as America.

Three-time Pulitzer Prize winner Thomas L. Friedman addressed the American conservatives' misconception about what it means to have free healthcare for all in Denmark.[192] Denmark is far from being a socialist-planned economy. It is a hypercompetitive market economy that has produced some of the most globally competitive multinationals in the world.

The US healthcare system should be changed radically to a publicly financed system like in Europe. It will be extremely difficult to accomplish such a change in a country where Trump got almost half of the votes for reelection after he had made more than 20,000 false or misleading claims during his presidency.[193]

Presidential campaigns are particularly malicious. In 2008, Republican vice-presidential candidate Sarah Palin established a new low, a tradition that everything could be used, no matter how hateful, spiteful, and mendacious it was, and regardless of whether the accusations were not even directed against the candidate, but a family member, a friend, a remote acquaintance, or were postulated to have happened in elementary school.[194]

In such a country, it is impossible for voters to vote rationally for what is best for themselves. Therefore, without ensuring a minimum level of honesty, America will not change. Trump propagated his lies about a rigged election until the very end and instilled so much hatred in his supporters that armed rioters stormed the halls of Congress to block Joe Biden's win on January 6, 2021.[195] Five people were killed, including a police officer murdered by the mob. Hours after he had ignited the riot, Trump finally called on his supporters to "go home" but spent a large amount of time in the one-minute video lamenting and lying about his election loss. In the evening, Trump justified the mob's actions and praised them in a tweet, which was deleted by Twitter. This is the worst we have ever seen happening in America. An attack on democracy itself.

Most Americans have European ancestors, and many Europeans have American friends and are very concerned about what we are witnessing. We would love to help, and I have this advice:

I do not advocate censorship, but America needs to tighten its libel laws substantially in relation to spreading malicious and blatant lies and hate speech. Some US hate speech preachers have been denied entry into many European countries. In order to establish a well-functioning, publicly funded healthcare, the culture needs to change radically, which cannot happen without introducing stiff penalties that include long jail sentences. This is justified because, as we have seen during the COVID-19 pandemic, lies can be deadly.

6

Human Papilloma Virus (HPV)

I have explained in previous chapters how I have come to the conclusions that everyone should get vaccinated against measles, whereas no one needs to get vaccinated against influenza.

The HPV vaccine is much more difficult. There are many uncertainties, both in relation to the benefits and to the harms. Unfortunately, the public debate has become polarized to the extreme and oversimplified, often reduced to whether you are for or against the vaccine even though the only thing you did was to ask a reasonable question.

My first encounter with the HPV vaccine was in 2008. Upon our eldest daughter's 12th birthday, we received a letter from a doctor asking us to enroll her in an HPV vaccine trial conducted by GlaxoSmithKline.[1] I asked to see the trial protocol, and after having read it, I alerted him to two issues:

There is nothing about harmful effects in the 105-page protocol, only some non-informative comments like "generally safe and well-tolerated." The readers are referred to the *Investigator's Brochure* about this. In the parents' information you can read that the vaccine has "affected the nervous system, blood cells, the thyroid and the kidneys." It would be relevant for us to know what that means and the frequencies of such potentially serious harms. If this information is included in the *Investigator's Brochure*, hopefully, it would be possible to hand it over to us. You cannot make an informed choice if you do not get statistics on the adverse effects.

It appears on pages 79–83 in the protocol that Glaxo owns the data and the investigators do not have any realistic possibilities of publishing the trial without the company's permission, among other things, because the company

must approve publications and because individual investigators will not gain
access to all data from the trial—only their own data.

I encouraged my colleague to ensure that the trial would be published no
matter what the results showed.

He responded that, unfortunately, it was not possible for him to send
me the *Investigator's Brochure*. He did not explain why.

We did not accept these conditions. The harms looked serious, but we
could not get relevant information about them. Furthermore, even that far
back, thousands of reports had been submitted to the authorities of serious
adverse events, including a few deaths.

In August 2015, I declined an invitation to a meeting about possible
harms of the HPV vaccine at the Danish Board of Health, as I had no particular interest in this vaccine. However, the former head of Cabinet in the
Ministry of Health convinced me to come, hoping I would find there was
no reason to worry about the safety of the vaccine.

The opposite happened. What impressed me the most was a lecture
by Dr. Louise Brinth from the Danish Syncope Unit, who had seen many
of the affected girls—predominantly elite sportswomen. Such people have
weakened immune defenses because stress hormones weaken immune
responses. It therefore made sense that, if something went awry after vaccination, it might primarily affect such women. Most patients at the Unit had
been elderly, but now many were girls or young women.[2]

It was suspected that the HPV vaccine might cause serious neurological disorders, one of which is postural orthostatic tachycardia syndrome
(POTS), in which a change from lying to standing causes an abnormally
large increase in heart rate that may be accompanied by light-headedness,
trouble thinking, blurred vision, and weakness. Another is chronic regional
pain syndrome (CRPS).

Denmark contacted the European Commission with its concerns, and
in July 2015, the EMA was asked to assess the research linking the HPV
vaccine to serious harms.[3] This research included three papers published by
Brinth and coworkers.[4] She had studied a consecutive cohort of 75 patients
referred to the Syncope Unit for a head-up tilt test due to orthostatic intolerance and symptoms compatible with autonomic dysfunction as a suspected
adverse effect following vaccination. She excluded 11 patients because the
onset of symptoms was later than the first two postvaccination months: 7
with known chronic diseases or in whom other possible eliciting factors

could be recognized and 4 who were unable to account for the temporal association between vaccination and symptom onset.

The most common symptoms in the remaining 53 patients were headache (100%), orthostatic intolerance (96%), fatigue (96%), nausea (91%), cognitive dysfunction (89%), disordered sleep (85%), feeling bloated (77%), hypersensitivity to light or blurred vision (70%), abdominal pain (70%), involuntary muscle activity in the form of intermittent tremor and myoclonic twitches (66%), neuropathic pain (66%), and muscle weakness in the extremities (57%).[5] In six cases, the muscle weakness led to disablement with very limited walking distances and confinement to a wheelchair for longer periods of time. All but one (98%) reported that their activities of daily living were seriously affected, and 75% had had to quit school or work for more than two months.

Symptoms of dysautonomia are diffuse and widespread because the autonomic nervous system innervates, monitors, and controls most of the tissues and organs in the body.[6] Brinth argued that POTS should probably be considered a symptom secondary to another, yet unidentified, condition rather than as a disease entity of its own.

When large numbers of people are vaccinated, some of them might develop autoimmune disorders, e.g., narcolepsy after flu shots (see Chapter 4). If the HPV vaccine causes dysautonomia, we would expect to find autoantibodies against the autonomic nervous system. In one study, such autoantibodies were found in most of 17 patients with POTS, whereas 7 patients with vasovagal syncope and 11 healthy controls did not have them.[7] Another, larger study was carried out at the Danish Syncope Centre. It showed that, after vaccination, autoantibodies were identified in most girls with POTS combined with other symptoms of dysautonomia, but only in a minority of those vaccinated girls who were healthy, and in even fewer healthy controls.[8] There are additional such studies.[9]

Brinth interpreted her study of the symptoms after vaccination cautiously and did not claim a causal relationship.[10] She identified POTS in 60% of the patients[11] and found that 87% and 90% of the patients fulfilled the official criteria for chronic fatigue syndrome (CFS) and myalgic encephalomyelitis (ME), respectively.[12]

* * *

In its submission to EMA, the Danish Health and Medicines Authorities also included a review of the global adverse events data on the HPV vaccines made by the Uppsala Monitoring Centre, a WHO collaborating center that accepts reports of suspected harms of vaccines and other drugs.

EMA worked fast. Already in November 2015, EMA issued a 40-page report concluding that "the evidence does not support a causal association between HPV vaccination and CRPS and/or POTS" and that "The benefits of HPV vaccines continue to outweigh their risks."[13] Thus, the message was that there was nothing to worry about.

The report also stated that the safety of the vaccines should continue to be carefully monitored, which is a standard clause that exonerates the authorities should it later turn out that they overlooked something. The media triumphantly touted that the case was settled for good and were very aggressive toward Brinth and her colleagues. The headline in a major Danish newspaper ran: "Danish researchers knocked down: No correlation between HPV vaccine and severe symptoms. The European Medicines Agency strongly criticises Danish researchers' methods."[14]

This article ignited a witch hunt,[15] although Brinth had only done what every doctor should do—report her observations—which is how we gain new knowledge. I can see nothing wrong with her methods, but the newspaper referred uncritically to EMA's assertion that "Overall, the case series reported by Brinth and colleagues (2015) is considered to represent a highly selected sample of patients, apparently chosen to fit a pre-specified hypothesis of vaccine-induced injury."[16]

EMA's statement was outrageous and wrong. Brinth had included all consecutively referred patients,[17] except those that did not meet the inclusion criteria, and EMA's allegations constituted guesswork ("apparently") and came close to an accusation of scientific misconduct. Furthermore, as Brinth's studies led to a hypothesis of vaccine-induced harms, it excludes the possibility that patients were selected to fit a prespecified hypothesis.

The newspaper had asked Leif Vestergaard, director of the Danish Cancer Society, if he thought Brinth's research bordered on scientific misconduct. He said that others should make this judgment but added that EMA had raised a very serious criticism.

What is "very serious" is that EMA wrote as it did, and that Vestergaard willingly contributed to the witch hunt. Few researchers would be willing to communicate their suspicions about possible harms of drugs if they knew they might risk such harassment and humiliation. Brinth has suffered tremendously,[18] and her children have been harassed at school. It's unbelievable, but the mentality of the Inquisition will be with us forever.

Vestergaard did not pull any punches but called for the National Board of Health to investigate whether clinics like the Syncope Centre had the right staff. This is typical when the Empire strikes back: "We remove critical voices but won't say so directly."

However, in another article the same day, Liselott Blixt, chair of the Health Committee in Parliament, stated: "I don't trust the group that made the report. I always thought the wrong people were asked to investigate this. Most of them are or have been on the payroll of vaccine manufacturers. They are very biased."[19] She added that she felt the Syncope Centre was the most credible part in the debate and that they didn't say they wanted to stop the vaccine but only pointed out that they received a lot of sick girls and that there might be a connection. So true, but witch hunters don't care about the truth.

Critical journalism has become difficult because of the increasing concentration of the money in rather few corporations that exert an enormous influence on politics. I have experienced several times that editors have suddenly scrapped interviews with me that their journalists had carefully written up and that were very relevant. I found out every time that these media had been corrupted by industry money or were highly dependent on the income from drug advertisements.

HPV vaccines are no exception. Danish journalists have written about an industry that surveys the journalists' research, spreads doubt about their sources, spreads fear, and intimidates.[20] A journalist working on a story about a girl who quit school after experiencing serious harms of the HPV vaccine was contacted by Mads Damkjær, senior market access manager at Sanofi Pasteur MSD, before the story was printed. Damkjær tried to convince him that the girl was an unreliable source. Some doctors mentioned a brochure that discussed the benefits from the vaccination. It was available in the offices of family physicians and was written by a doctor on Sanofi's payroll, but they all declined to be interviewed because they were afraid of Sanofi.

Another journalist contacted the Danish Board of Health to get an interview about the possible harms of the HPV vaccine, but the next day she was contacted by a woman from a PR agency that worked for Sanofi who said she knew what the journalist was working on. She consistently described side effect as "rumors" or "myths," which originated from America's powerful but totally untrustworthy anti-vaccine lobby.

The same day the journalist published her article, Damkjær complained to the editor that she was a "horny frontpage seeking impossible person" who "reads numbers and facts like Satan reads the Bible," and he added that

Danish media were so pressured that one could feed pigs with unemployed journalists, and that a catastrophe like her did not have diligence, fairness, or source criticism among her virtues.

The journalist noted that doctors who had communicated their concerns to the authorities were unwilling to be interviewed for fear of damaging their relationship with the industry and of being associated with anti-vaccine radicalized "idiots."

Damkjær opined that the critical journalism meant that five of the 1,300 girls who would not be vaccinated would die. This says something about Sanofi's way of dealing with numbers. See also next how Sanofi avoided to detect POTS in its database.

EMA's Poor Job with Assessing the Harms of the Vaccines

As noted, EMA published a 40-page report in November 2015 concluding that there are no serious neurological harms of the HPV vaccines.[21] We wanted to submit a complaint over maladministration to the European Ombudsman, but according to the rules, we first needed to complain to EMA itself.

In May 2016, we submitted a 19-page complaint[22] in which we also commented on a leaked confidential report used to brief EMA's appointed scientific advisory group.[23] This 256-page "briefing note to experts" was stamped *Confidential* across every page. It shows that there were important disagreements between the experts, suggesting more uncertainty in the science than EMA's official report revealed.[24]

EMA Trusted the Manufacturers to Report Reliably on Harms

EMA's replies to us were disappointing. Some of our concerns were not addressed, and several statements were incorrect or seriously misleading. We have published our most important observations.[25]

Despite numerous scandals where concealment of serious harms has led to hundreds of thousands of patients dying unnecessarily,[26] drug regulators still trust the drug companies. EMA asked the manufacturers to evaluate whether their vaccines are safe, review cases of CRPS and POTS in their trials, go through their postmarketing surveillance data, use these data to produce "observed versus expected" analyses of adverse events, and review and assess the published scientific literature.[27]

Weaknesses in the scientific strategy employed by the companies were obvious. EMA's official report[28] did not mention that the search strategies the manufacturers used to search their databases were inadequate[29] and must have overlooked many cases.[30] The companies did not search for *headache* even though all of Brinth's patients had headaches, and *dizziness* needed to occur together with *orthostatic intolerance* or *orthostatic heart rate response increased* in order to count. EMA nonetheless uncritically reproduced the incidence rates of CRPS and POTS constructed by the manufacturers.[31]

Industry-run searches prior to EMA's review had also been inadequate. In 2014, the Danish drug regulator instructed Sanofi Pasteur MSD, which manufactures Gardasil, one of the HPV vaccines, on how to search specific symptoms in its database including dizziness, palpitations, rapid heart rate, tremor, fatigue, and fainting. Despite these clear instructions, Sanofi only searched *postural dizziness, orthostatic intolerance*, and *palpitations and dizziness*. The Danish authorities discovered this because only 3 of 26 registered Danish reports of POTS showed up in Sanofi's searches.[32]

EMA knew it could not trust the drug companies. A colleague provided us with a copy of an expert assessment report for Gardasil 9, the nine-valent version of Gardasil, written on behalf of EMA.[33] The rapporteurs were concerned that Sanofi had avoided identifying possible cases of serious harms of the vaccine. Their concerns were shared by EMA's own trial inspectors,[34] who criticized that adverse events were only reported for 14 days after each vaccination; that any new symptoms at other times were reported as "new medical events" without medical assessments or final outcomes being recorded; and that the reporting of serious adverse events was not required during the full course of the trial even though systemic side effects could appear long after the vaccinations were given.[35] The inspectors also criticized that three people had been diagnosed with POTS in the clinical safety database after receipt of Gardasil 9 but that these were not reported as adverse events; that a case of POTS after Gardasil was called "new medical history" instead of an adverse event; that hospitalization for severe dizziness was not reported as a serious adverse event; and that for another person the term *dysautonomia* was not included on the list of events.

The criticism is very serious, and an investigative journalist at *Slate* made similar observations.[36] He described three Danish women who experienced serious adverse events after Gardasil in a clinical trial, but their complaints were never registered as adverse events, which they should have been. When the journalist contacted the investigator handling two of the cases, Dr. Anette Kjærbye-Thygesen at Hvidovre Hospital, she declined to be interviewed. The hospital's press officer wrote in an email that "Regarding registration of various symptoms and health data, the doctor states that she has followed the trial protocol."[37] The hospital also declined to address his questions.

One of the three women had brought up her symptoms with study personnel at every visit during the four-year trial and even told them her illness had forced her to quit school. But no one took her seriously. They kept saying: "This is not the kind of side effects we see with this vaccine."

Numerous such omissions occurred. Brinth told me about them, which she learned from a colleague who was an investigator in a trial.

While Merck says otherwise, there is no indication in its confidential study protocol that it would use "new medical history" as a safety metric.[38] And it would not have worked: the worksheet allotted just one line per entry, with no measurement of symptom severity, duration, outcome, or seriousness (a serious adverse event is one that results in death, is life-threatening, requires hospitalization or prolongation of existing hospitalization, results in persistent or significant disability, or is a congenital anomaly or birth defect).

I have never heard of safety data being collected in this way. Any new finding should automatically have triggered an adverse event report. A press officer from the Danish Medicines Agency, which approved Merck's Future 2 protocol in 2002, pointed out that it contained no mention of "new medical history" or "new medical conditions." In an email, the press officer wrote, "We are also not aware of whether this category has been used in other clinical trials with drugs, as these are not terms that are used according to guidelines."[39]

A drug-safety adviser at a multinational pharmaceutical company told the *Slate* journalist that "Everything from the first injection to the last plus a follow-up period is what we call treatment-emergent adverse events." She puzzled over the brief, interrupted follow-up periods in the Gardasil trials (only 14 days), as well as Merck's choice not to report nonserious adverse events for all participants and its dismissal of many events as medical history. "This is completely bonkers," the drug-safety adviser said, requesting not to be named for fear of compromising her position in the industry.[40]

In their final report recommending conditional approval of Gardasil 9, the EMA rapporteurs asked Merck to "discuss the impact of [its] unconventional and potentially suboptimal method of reporting adverse events and provide reassurance on the overall completeness and accuracy of safety data provided in the application."[41] However, in EMA's publicly available assessment of Gardasil 9, all mention of the safety concerns had been scrubbed.[42]

The journalist contacted Dr. Susanne Krüger Kjær, a professor from the Danish Cancer Society who oversaw the Danish part of Future 2, but she also declined to address the safety concerns: "I can't answer any of those questions because I didn't design the trial." However, she is responsible for it, being one of the authors on the trial report, which appeared in 2007 in the *New England Journal of Medicine* and contains no mention of "new medical history."[43]

No Placebo Controls in the Trials

There were other grave impediments to the assessment of serious harms of the vaccines. EMA allowed the manufacturers to lump what was misleadingly called the placebo groups in their trials. We complained to the European Ombudsman in October, 2016,[44] and in the ensuing correspondence, EMA Executive Director Guido Rasi explained to the Ombudsman that "all studies submitted for the marketing authorisation application for Gardasil were placebo controlled."[45] EMA's official report also gives this impression and mentions "placebo cohorts" for the Gardasil trials, and "a comparator group (either placebo or another vaccine)" for the Cervarix trials.[46] In the briefing note, EMA wrote about the potential association between the vaccine and CRPS, that the few cases reported from the randomized clinical trials were "evenly distributed between the qHPV and placebo groups which does not suggest an association."[47] EMA concluded the same for POTS: "The few cases reported from RCTs do not suggest an imbalance between the qHPV and placebo groups and does not suggest an association."[48]

We felt the drug companies and EMA had committed scientific misconduct and said so in our complaint to EMA,[49] as none of these comparisons were against placebo; they were against another vaccine or a vaccine adjuvant (which is a substance used to boost the immune response to a vaccine).

Not a single trial was truly placebo- (i.e., saline-) controlled.[50] In one Gardasil trial, 597 children received a so-called placebo, which included all the excipients in the carrier solution. In a Gardasil 9 trial, 306 participants received a saline placebo, but as they had all been vaccinated with Gardasil earlier,[51] those who did not tolerate Gardasil were likely not enrolled in the study. In the other Gardasil trials, the control group received a strongly immunogenic adjuvant, Amorphous Aluminium Hydroxyphosphate Sulfate (AAHS), $AlHO_9PS^{-3}$.

In the trials of Cervarix (GlaxoSmithKline), the control group received a vaccine against hepatitis A or B,[52] which contains an aluminium adjuvant similar to that in the company's HPV vaccines, or only the adjuvant, $Al(OH)_3$.

The use of active comparators may make it impossible to detect serious harms of the HPV vaccines in the randomized trials if the comparators cause similar harms. EMA did not address this fundamental flaw in its official report,[53] but it was brought up by two doctors external to EMA's expert group in the secret briefing note.[54] These doctors explained that Gardasil was initially compared with a placebo group, whereby the number of adverse reactions was much higher and more serious than in the control group. After comparing with 320 patients in the saline placebo group, a quick move was made to an aluminium-containing placebo, which distorted the comparison. Furthermore, no one would voluntarily want to be vaccinated with a toxic adjuvant, which was not necessary, as they could get a harmless saline solution. The doctors referred to Merck's package insert when saying that the differences between Gardasil and saline were noticeable. They furthermore showed two tables from the package insert and noted that the saline placebo only appeared separately in the table of local reactions on the injection site, whereas for serious adverse reactions, the saline and the adjuvant groups had been combined, "perhaps to cover up the major differences between these two groups."

WHO has stated that using adjuvant or another vaccine as comparator instead of placebo makes it difficult to assess the harms of a vaccine and that placebo can be used in trials of vaccines against diseases for which there are no existing vaccines.[55]

Because the HPV vaccines and their adjuvants[56] had similar harm profiles, the manufacturers and regulators concluded that the vaccines are safe. This is like saying that cigarettes and cigars must be safe because they have similar harm profiles.[57]

The FDA-approved package insert for Gardasil is highly revealing.[58] It confirms Brinth's observation that the most common adverse reaction is headache. It furthermore mentions that other common adverse reactions (frequency of at least 1.0% and greater than in the AAHS [aluminium adjuvant] control or saline placebo groups) are fever, nausea, and dizziness; and pain, swelling, erythema, pruritus, and bruising at the injection site. Quite a collection of harms, above those in the controls, considering that patients in the control groups were also harmed.

Merck writes about 18,083 people who participated in seven clinical trials where the control group received AAHS (five trials) or saline placebo (one trial) while the last study had no control group. They received the injections on the day of enrollment, and after approximately 2 and 6 months, and, as already noted, safety was evaluated for 14 days after each injection.

Table 1 in the package insert shows that Gardasil causes more local reactions than the adjuvant, which causes more local reactions than the saline placebo (and Table 4 shows that they are more severe, as well):

Table 1: Injection-Site Adverse Reactions in Girls and Women 9 Through 26 Years of Age*

Adverse Reaction (1 to 5 Days Postvaccination)	GARDASIL (N = 5088) %	AAHS Control[†] (N = 3470) %	Saline Placebo (N = 320) %
Injection Site			
Pain	83.9	75.4	48.6
Swelling	25.4	15.8	7.3
Erythema	24.7	18.4	12.1
Pruritus	3.2	2.8	0.6
Bruising	2.8	3.2	1.6

*The injection-site adverse reactions that were observed among recipients of GARDASIL were at a frequency of at least 1.0% and also at a greater frequency than that observed among AAHS control or saline placebo recipients.
[†]AAHS Control = Amorphous Aluminum Hydroxyphosphate Sulfate

If the control group had not received any injection, there would not have been any "local reactions at the injection site" to report. Thus, it is inappropriate to lump the two control groups, but in all tables of systemic adverse events, this was what Merck did.

Headache was the most commonly reported systemic adverse reaction, 28.2% with Gardasil and 28.4% with "AAHS control or saline placebo." Fever was the next most commonly reported systemic adverse reaction, 13.0% versus 11.2%. I don't believe that over 10% of girls and women 9 to 26 years of age would have gotten fever in a random 14-day period if they had not received a vaccine or vaccine adjuvant. The almost identical percentages therefore tell us that adjuvants are not safe.

Merck's reporting of serious adverse reactions is extremely misleading: "Serious Adverse Reactions in the Entire Study Population across the Clinical Studies, 258 individuals (GARDASIL N = 128 or 0.8%; placebo N = 130 or 1.0%) out of 29,323 (GARDASIL N = 15,706; AAHS control N = 13,023; or saline placebo N = 594)." This sentence is difficult to comprehend, and there were not 130 reactions on placebo because 130/594 =

22%, and not 1.0%, and what Merck calls placebo also includes the group that received the adjuvant.

Deaths were reported similarly misleadingly, as if there had been 19 deaths on placebo, but most of the "placebo" was the adjuvant. The death rate was 0.1%, both in the Gardasil group and in the adjuvant/placebo group.

There were also tables of systemic autoimmune disorders, which occurred in 2.3% versus 2.3% of the females, and in 1.5% versus 1.5% in males. It is totally inappropriate to record systemic autoimmune disorders only within 14 days after the third vaccination, as they may take much longer to develop or become diagnosed. Deaths could also occur later. Apart from this, I wonder why so many people developed systemic autoimmune disorders in such a short time.

It is unbelievable that FDA let Merck get away with information that is so misleading and with trials that only registered serious events in 14-day periods.

We Know Very Little about the Harms of Vaccine Adjuvants

In an email to the Ombudsman, EMA's Director Guido Rasi stated that the aluminium adjuvants are safe, that their use has been established for several decades, and that the substances are defined in the European Pharmacopoeia.[59] Rasi also mentioned that the assessment of the evidence for the safety of the adjuvants had been performed over many years by EMA and other health authorities, such as the European Food Safety Authority, FDA, and WHO. He gave references to all of the authorities, but none of them supported his claim about safety.

Three links, to EMA, FDA, and WHO, were all dead.[60] One worked two years later but contained nothing of relevance. The link to the European Food Safety Authority was about safety of aluminium from dietary intake, which has nothing to do with aluminium adjuvants in vaccines. The intestinal absorption of aluminium is very poor, and almost all absorbed aluminium is excreted from the body.

The last link was to a WHO report where a Global Advisory Committee on Vaccine Safety (GACVS) wrote 280 words about aluminium adjuvants.[61] GACVS reviewed two published studies alleging that aluminium in vaccines is associated with autism spectrum disorders and concluded that these two studies were seriously flawed. GACVS also reviewed the evidence generated from two FDA risk assessment models of aluminium-containing vaccines. The FDA indicated that the body burden of aluminium following injections of aluminium-containing vaccines never exceeds US regulatory safety thresholds based on orally ingested aluminium. Rasi's quote of the GACVS report is misleading, as it confuses orally ingested aluminium with the effect of parenteral aluminium in an adjuvant. Furthermore, clinical effects are not likely to reflect the dose of the metal, aluminium, but the immunogenicity, which is the reason to administer the adjuvant.[62] In contrast to Rasi's assertions about the European Pharmacopoeia, the properties of the aluminium adjuvants are not well defined. Rasi gives the impression that the aluminium adjuvants in the HPV vaccines are similar to those used since 1926.[63] However, the Gardasil adjuvant is amorphous aluminium hydroxyphosphate sulfate, $AlHO_9PS^{-3}$, or AAHS, which have other properties than aluminium hydroxide, which is the substance Rasi mentions.

We have investigated whether the safety of AAHS has ever been tested in comparison with an inert substance in humans. We have been unable to find any evidence of this. Merck's AAHS has a confidential formula; its properties are variable from batch to batch and even within batches.[64] The harms caused by the adjuvant are therefore likely to vary.

For aluminium hydroxide, human and animal studies have shown harms. In a large randomized trial in humans, influenza vaccines caused 34% more adverse events when they contained adjuvant than when they did not, risk ratio 1.34 (1.23 to 1.45, p < 0.0001) and also more severe adverse events, risk ratio 2.71 (1.65 to 4.44, p < 0.0001) (my calculations).[65] These adverse events were recorded up to only three days after the vaccination.

The few studies that have been carried out on aluminium hydroxide and similar adjuvants are vastly insufficient. One study, for example, included only two rabbits per adjuvant, and the follow-up was too short to find out what happened to the aluminium that was not excreted, which was most of the injected amount.[66]

Editorial Misconduct in Animal Study of Aluminium Hydroxide Adjuvant

Farmers had observed serious behavioral changes in sheep vaccinated against bluetongue disease,[67] which were confirmed in an experimental study in 2013.[68] Animal studies have shown severe meningoencephalitis and neuronal necrosis on autopsy, and in mice, transport of aluminium from the injection site to the central nervous system has been demonstrated after injections with aluminium hydroxide adjuvant.[69]

A subsequent study showed that, compared to placebo, sheep injected repeatedly with the adjuvant or the vaccine had fewer affiliative interactions and increases in aggressive interactions, stereotypies, excitatory behavior, and compulsive eating.[70] The study was published in *Pharmacological Research* on November 3, 2018 (as an e-publication online first), but has been retracted by the editor and can no longer be found on the journal's website.[71]

I have a copy of the retracted study and have corresponded with the lead author, Lluís Luján. It is a case of serious editorial misconduct, which might have involved a troll financed by a vaccine manufacturer.

The editor-in-chief, Professor Emilio Clementi, wrote to Luján on January 11, 2019, that he had "received serious concerns from the readership," which he detailed but without revealing the source, which seems to be only one person. Clementi asked Luján if he wanted to withdraw the manuscript.

Luján replied that he did not understand why the complainant was anonymous and that he would respond to the concerns. He also offered to make the raw data available for independent statistical analysis and noted that there are people who write to editors of papers that question the safety of vaccines.

A little later, Luján wrote that the comments had almost no scientific foundation but were written to deceive and to give the appearance of "scientific credibility." He knew about authors having received similar "complaints" where the objective was to get a published paper retracted and to discredit the authors' reputation. Most of these "complaints" came from a few sources that rarely—if ever—revealed their conflicts of interest.

Luján used seven pages to rebutt the concerns raised, and his discussion of the issues is convincing. The "concerned reader" had made numerous elementary errors.

Next, Clementi asked his statistical editor, Professor Elia Biganzoli, to look at the issues. He advised against withdrawal of the paper and noted that its limitations were common in animal studies. He suggested that additional research be carried out to clarify the role of vaccines and the adjuvant; noted that Luján and coworkers regarded their results as preliminary; called for an editorial to accompany the paper; and noted that the criticism was possibly biased by advocacy, "which is a disgraceful attitude in science."

This was clearly the best way forward. Allowing open scientific debate is what furthers science. However, six days later, on February 19, Clementi wrote to Luján that he would withdraw the paper while allowing him to resubmit a revised version that took into account the criticisms raised by his statistical editor, and which would then be assessed for possible publication.

When editors write like this, it is virtually certain that they will reject the paper after resubmission and are merely looking for an excuse to do so.

Luján responded that this was unjustified, as he had addressed all "concerns" and had not had a chance to respond to the statistical review, after which he provided a rebuttal of Biganzoli's arguments.

Anne Marie Pordon from Elsevier, the publisher of the journal, wrote that the manuscript was not being retracted, "which implies wrongdoing and could damage your professional reputation. We are withdrawing the paper, which does not imply misconduct in any way. There will be simply a statement that says 'This paper has been withdrawn at the request of the _____' (Authors or Editors in the blank)."

This is nonsense. There is no difference between withdrawal and retraction, and Elsevier uses both words in its policy statement, as you will soon see. It is also like saying: "Do you wish to commit professional suicide, or do you prefer we do it for you?"

Luján responded that criticism of a published paper should appear in a Letter to the Editor in a published issue of the journal and that he could only accept his publication in its present form. He noted that most complaints came from David Hawkes or some of his accomplices who were paid by the vaccine industry to contest any published paper where there might be any suggestion that a vaccine is not 100% safe. The reason why Luján suspected that David Hawkes was the anonymous complainant is that Benzoli had suggested it would be relevant to cite a systematic review by him about the scientific basis for the creation of a new syndrome, Autoimmune Syndrome Induced by Adjuvants (ASIA).[72]

On the journal's website, the article is mentioned this way: "This article has been withdrawn at the request of the editor. The Publisher apologizes for any inconvenience this may cause."[73] There was no explanation whatsoever but a link, "Download full text in PDF." Naively, I thought I could find the withdrawn article there, but it was gone. The only thing the link showed was this:

WITHDRAWN: Cognition and behavior in sheep repetitively inoculated with
aluminum adjuvant-containing vaccines or aluminum adjuvant only

Javier Asín[a,1], María Pascual-Alonso[b,1], Pedro Pinczowski[a], Marina Gimeno[a], Marta Pérez[c,d],
Ana Muniesa[a,d], Lorena de Pablo-Maiso[e], Ignacio de Blas[a,d], Delia Lacasta[a,d],
Antonio Fernández[a,d], Damián de Andrés[e], Gustavo María[b,d], Ramsés Reina[e,2], Lluís Luján[a,d,2,*]

[a] Department of Animal Pathology, University of Zaragoza, Spain
[b] Department of Animal Production and Food Science, University of Zaragoza, Spain
[c] Department of Anatomy, Embryology and Animal Genetics, University of Zaragoza, Spain
[d] Instituto Universitario de Investigación Mixto Agroalimentario de Aragón (IA2), University of Zaragoza, Spain
[e] Institute of Agrobiotechnology, CSIC-Public University of Navarra, Mutilva Baja, Navarra, Spain

Elsevier's policy on article withdrawal states that an article accepted for publication can be withdrawn if it includes errors, duplicates another article, or
violates ethics guidelines (e.g., by bogus claims of authorship or fraud).

Elsevier violated its own rules. Not only did none of the reasons for
withdrawal apply, but this rule was also ignored: "The original article is
retained unchanged save for a watermark on the .pdf indicating on each
page that it is 'retracted.'"

Elsevier also violated the guidelines established by the Committee on
Publication Ethics (COPE) even though Elsevier is a member of COPE:
"Notices of retraction should . . . state the reason(s) for retraction (to distin-
guish misconduct from honest error)."[74]

The prestigious International Committee of Medical Journal Editors
notes: "The text of the retraction should explain why the article is being
retracted and include a complete citation reference to that article. Retracted
articles should remain in the public domain and be clearly labelled as
retracted."[75]

I consider this whole affair editorial misconduct of the worst kind. No
fairness, no explanation, and no article. It is outrageous that this could
happen. Elsevier is one of the wealthiest publishers in the world, which is
because they charge exorbitant prices, also for subscriptions by university
libraries.[76] We should not publish in Elsevier journals. Lancet, which protected Wakefield (see Chapter 2), is also an Elsevier journal.

Medical journals have a parasitic relationship with researchers.
Researchers do research that is often publicly funded, write it up, and publish it, and other researchers and public institutions then need to pay for
access. Furthermore, researchers do peer review of submitted articles for
free. There is growing criticism of this arrangement, and some researchers
establish their own journals to avoid the exhortation and to make their

articles available at an affordable price, or for free. In 2012, the faculty at Harvard University wrote that some journals cost as much as $40,000 per year and that prices for online content from two providers had increased by about 145% over six years.[77]

EMA Concealed Its Literature Searches for Its Own Experts

EMA mentioned in its confidential briefing note to experts that it had done systematic literature searches for POTS and CRPS.[78] There were brief descriptions of what EMA had found (less than a page for each syndrome), but just above these descriptions, there were statements that confidential information had been removed:

European Medicines Agency

- **HPV referral – literature search POTS**

   The EMA has performed a systematic bibliographic search regarding Postural Orthostatic Tachycardia Syndrome:

   [Confidential information was removed]

I later found out that there was nothing "confidential" in this information. In another internal EMA report,[79] the information about EMA's searches was blackened out before EMA released the document to a requester:

European Medicines Agency

- **HPV referral – litterature search POTS**

   The EMA has performed a systematic bibliographic search regarding Postural Orthostatic Tachycardia Syndrome:

In his letter to the Ombudsman, Rasi claimed that "said icon was inadvertently deleted further to a clerical error."[80] We found it hard to believe that clerical errors could explain that two icons, one for POTS and one for CRPS, were deleted in one document and that "Confidential information was removed" in another. It seemed deliberate that EMA did not want to share the results of its literature searches with its experts or with the public in case people asked for access to the confidential documents.

When I asked EMA's deputy director, Noël Wathion, to explain how this could possibly have happened, he did not reply.

The Ombudsman also found this problematic and encouraged us to obtain the missing literature searches from EMA, which we did. It turned out that a lot more was missing than just the search strategies. The blackened-out icons revealed that two Word documents were missing, one of which was for POTS:

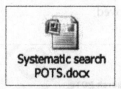

We received 14 pages with 15 references, which are highly relevant to the question of whether HPV vaccines or other vaccines may cause POTS or CRPS,[81] e.g., this statement: "POTS . . . frequently start after viral illness."[82] This is what I had suspected could happen and why I find it unacceptable that the "placebo" in the trials was another vaccine or the adjuvant. The changes in the immune system elicited by strongly immunogenic vaccines or adjuvants could render the vaccinated women more susceptible to the development of POTS or CRPS after an otherwise harmless viral illness. In the briefing note, EMA did actually mention that "Benarroch found that up to 50% of cases have antecedent of viral illness,"[83] but we missed this important information because it appeared under a discussion about how the companies had defined POTS.

The Ombudsman wrote to us that essentially all publications identified by EMA were included in the list of references available to the experts and that a summary of the results of the literature search was made available to them.[84] However, whether publications are listed or not doesn't matter. What matters is whether EMA left out important information from its literature searches in its two summaries in the briefing note, which it did.

EMA's literature searches showed that chronic fatigue syndrome has been linked to other vaccines and vaccine adjuvants; that some of the POTS patients might have small-fiber neuropathy; that there were case reports of CRPS after other vaccines (including hepatitis B vaccine, which was used in the control groups in the Cervarix trials); and that autoantibodies were found in 33% of 82 CRPS patients and in only 4% of 90 healthy controls.[85]

EMA noted that the experts could have asked for the literature searches if they needed them. But the experts could not know that important information was missing in the 256-page report they received. Furthermore, few people would dare ask a drug regulator to give them something the regulator had removed because it was "confidential."

In response to our complaint, the Ombudsman suggested that EMA consider making publicly available lists of all relevant documents in its possession related to a specific referral procedure. "Unfortunately, EMA did not address this suggestion." The Ombudsman therefore repeated her suggestion when closing her inquiry.[86]

Observed versus Expected Incidence of Serious Harms

EMA's key argument, mentioned ten times in its official report,[87] was that there was no difference between what was observed and the expected background incidence in the manufacturers' analysis. However, the briefing note revealed that both the Belgian and the Swedish co-rapporteurs were critical of the observed versus expected analyses.[88] EMA's official report did not reflect the substantial doubts about these analyses, but it admitted that the underlying research is of such poor quality that such comparisons cannot confirm a causal relationship between vaccines and harms even if it existed.[89]

The Ombudsman's inquiry team "takes no view on the scientific aspects of this question. However, it notes that the explanations provided are logical and appear reasonable."[90] The Ombudsman was inconsistent, as she, on many occasions, trusted EMA's scientific assessments based on the data the drug companies gave them,[91] whereas she refused to take a view on our scientific criticism.

In some analyses, the observed incidence of chronic fatigue syndrome was used to estimate the expected incidence of POTS, which is inappropriate and likely led to an overestimate of the expected incidence and thus a reduced chance to detect a harms signal.[92] EMA noted that for POTS, the observed number of cases was generally *lower* than expected under almost all assumptions except for Denmark.[93] This observation should have alerted EMA to the fact that the analyses performed by the drug companies were unreliable and that the data from Denmark were likely more complete than data from other countries.

In one of the reports EMA withheld from its experts, EMA admitted that no data were available on the background incidence and prevalence of POTS.[94] This was also found in a 2017 literature review[95] and renders EMA's "observed versus expected" statements meaningless.

EMA Distrusted Independent Research

The Danish Health Authorities and the Uppsala Monitoring Centre, both of which had found signals of harm, were dissatisfied with how their observations and reports were dismissed by EMA.

EMA erroneously claimed that Brinth's studies included no objective clinical evaluation.[96] All her papers stated that the orthostatic intolerance was quantified through tilt-testing, which is the benchmark test for POTS. Furthermore, it was troubling that only 33 of 83 cases of POTS that Brinth had described were considered by the manufacturers, and therefore also EMA, to have met the case definition criteria.[97] An assessment provided by a clinical expert who sees the patients is likely more reliable than that performed by a company employee looking at paperwork. EMA's problematic exclusion of cases was criticized by the Danish authorities in the confidential EMA report,[98] and they also disagreed with EMA's assessment that "the finding of the majority of POTS cases in Denmark does not support a causal relationship."[99] This disagreement was not mentioned in the official report.[100] The rapporteur concluded in the briefing note about the Uppsala report that "the HPV case reports from Denmark are distinguished from those from other countries by the fact that they contain an increased amount of clinical information and that certain, specific diagnostic PTs [preferred terms] are more commonly used."[101] This important information was not mentioned in the official report.[102]

EMA did not find the submitted evidence from the Uppsala Centre important, although the center found that POTS was reported 82 times more often for HPV vaccines than for other vaccines.[103] The finding that substantially more cases were serious for the HPV vaccines was mentioned in the official report but not paid attention to, although 80% of POTS cases and 78% of chronic fatigue syndrome cases required hospital admission or resulted in disability or interruption of normal function.[104]

Key people at the Uppsala Centre considered that their data were disregarded by EMA without adequate justification.[105] In September 2016, they published a paper online that strengthened my suspicion that the HPV vaccines may cause serious harms.[106] For the largest clusters they identified in the WHO VigiBase(R), the combination of headache and dizziness with either fatigue or syncope was more commonly reported in HPV vaccine reports than in other vaccine reports for females aged 9–25 years, and this disproportionality remained when countries reporting the signals of CRPS (Japan) and POTS (Denmark) were excluded. Even though the researchers reduced the possible influence of media attention by including only cases reported before the media attention, they identified a greater number of potentially undiagnosed cases than the *total* number of cases labeled with one of these diagnoses by the drug companies.

Conflicts of Interest at EMA

Contrary to EMA's statements,[107] EMA's policy about preventing conflicted experts from participating in its review of the HPV vaccines was not correctly applied. There were no restrictions for the chair of the Scientific Advisory Group, Andrew Pollard, although he had declared several conflicts of interest in relation to the HPV vaccine manufacturers in his role as principal investigator. In contrast, some of the advisors who were restricted had no such conflicts of interest.[108] EMA's claim that none of the experts had financial interests that could affect their impartiality was also wrong, as some of them, in addition to Pollard, had financial ties to the vaccine manufacturers.[109]

The Ombudsman did not understand how medical researchers define conflicts of interest but wrote: "There is no evidence that the expert's previous research work established any form of dependence on the producers of HPV vaccines."[110] Whether this can be proven or not in the concrete case is irrelevant, and it is EMA's duty to adhere to its own rules, which it didn't.

We had a long-drawn correspondence with EMA after we found out that its executive director, Guido Rasi, had not declared that he is the inventor behind several patents.[111] As some of them were recent, we believed he should have declared them, according to EMA's own regulations.

If Rasi believed he didn't have a problem, he could have told us so. But he never contacted us. He involved a law firm and let his deputy, Noël Wathion, run an attack on us. In his first letter, Wathion wrote:

> EMA would like to refute your unsubstantiated allegations in the strongest
> possible terms . . . EMA staff members are required to declare in their decla-
> ration of interests (DoI) any ownership of a patent . . . An inventor . . . is not
> necessarily the owner . . . Prof Rasi does not own any patent together with

Sigma-Tau . . . He is not even the beneficiary of those patent families . . .
Taking into account the seriousness of the accusations made via the Internet
and the echo that these allegations have had worldwide, EMA reserves the
right to protect its reputation through all appropriate means.

I don't know what Wathion meant about spreading accusations via the
Internet. I am not aware any of us did that.

Three weeks later, Carter-Ruck solicitors in London wrote to us that
our comments about Rasi were "highly defamatory" and that he had never
had any economic rights or financial benefits from his patents. The lawyers
made it clear that Rasi did not wish to become embroiled in a legal dispute
but that he hoped we would agree "to amend the relevant passages of the
Publication, and to publish (in terms to be agreed) a suitable statement of
correction and apology withdrawing these false allegations."

We explained that it would be wrong to change published documents.
If errors are detected in scientific papers, the papers are not changed but
errata are published separately. We attached a document we aimed to
publish where we described the issues, apologized, and explained that we
were not aware of the legal subtleties and assumed that an inventor of a
patented technology is also an owner of that patent, as it is highly unusual
that inventors give away their patents to drug companies without benefiting
from them.

The lawyers wrote back that Rasi could not accept our wording and
sent a revised version, which was unacceptable to us because we were asked
to accept statements as facts, although we had no possibility of checking if
Rasi did not own the patents he had invented.

We also explained that an apology is a very personal thing, and that
a person asking for an apology should not require a particular text or for-
mat, as the apology would then not be genuine. Furthermore, we could not
accept that our explanation had been deleted, as we needed to protect our
own reputations by noting that our mistake was made in good faith. We
proposed that our apology should include: "Noël Wathion has explained to
us that Professor Rasi is not the owner of the patents for which he is named
as inventor."

We were convinced that this would settle the issue, but the law firm
responded that, rather that engage in further protracted correspondence,
they proposed a telephone discussion to try to resolve any remaining issues.
Given our experience with lawyers, we replied that we preferred to communicate in writing.

Next, the lawyers wanted us to include this sentence: "On the basis of these assurances we accept that Professor Rasi has never had, and does not have, any economic rights or financial interest or benefit (whether actual or potential) in, or arising from, any of the patents to which the Publication refers." We replied that lawyers know very well that, in court cases, one cannot force people to accept and declare what others tell them is the truth.

But the lawyers wouldn't give up. They tried again, this time starting with, "We acknowledge Mr Wathion's statement that . . ." We responded that Wathion had never made any such statement to us.

We then received the 8th letter from Rasi's lawyers explaining that Rasi had "no desire to engage further in protracted correspondence and mutual inconvenience." This ended a correspondence that had started almost three months earlier.

We found EMA's arguments untenable. Whatever the rules are, a top executive in an EU institution should ensure that not the slightest suspicion can be raised that he failed to declare his conflicts of interest. A rule of thumb is that if a normal person would be embarrassed if real or possible conflicts of interest were revealed that had not been declared, then it is wrong not to declare them. Rasi failed this simple and sensible test.

Another reason why it would have made sense for Rasi to declare his patents is that the public has so little confidence in the drug industry that it is similar to the confidence they have in tobacco companies and automobile repair shops.[112] Furthermore, people have been informed in newspaper articles and TV documentaries that corruption at the upper levels of drug agencies occurs.[113]

In response to our complaint over EMA, the Ombudsman noted that it would be wise to provide information about a staff member's prior ownership of patents and patent applications and asked EMA to strengthen its rules. As the Ombudsman's letter can no longer be found on her website, I have uploaded it on my own.[114]

Witch Hunt because of Our Complaint over EMA

Our complaint over EMA started a bizarre witch hunt by people in senior positions in Denmark who embarrassed themselves and their institutions by spreading blatantly false information in tweets and on Facebook.

It started with an e-letter published in March 2017 in a pretty unknown journal, *NPJ Vaccines*.[115] The web address to the letter begins with http://

www.nature.com, and some people believed it was published in the famous journal *Nature*, but *NPJ Vaccines* is just a *Nature* partner journal.

The letter's authors complained that we used the Nordic Cochrane Centre's letterhead when we wrote to EMA and the European Ombudsman. They argued that this gave the impression that our views were representative of, or were approved by, the Cochrane Collaboration. They lamented that this view was being promoted in online anti-vaccine communities. However, their two references did not support their claim, as it was clear and explicit in these articles that our criticism of EMA came from the Centre.

The authors wrote they had raised the matter with the Cochrane Steering Group that replied to them, but in their published e-letter they had left out these important bits of the reply: "The letter [to EMA] does not state that it was prepared on behalf of Cochrane and it is not an official statement of the Cochrane Collaboration . . . and, to our knowledge, they are using their correct affiliations."

Hence, this was a "noncase," and nothing should have come out of it. But influential people in Denmark abused the letter in the most spectacular fashion.

The director of the Danish Medicines Agency, Thomas Senderovitz, tweeted: "@PGtzschel's erroneous criticism of EMA's assessment of #HPV vaccine side effects on @CochraneNordic paper is problematic"[116] and "Precisely! Excellent post pointing out misinformation from Nordic Cochrane"[117] in response to a tweet by Karen Price: "How easy is misinformation???"[118] This was "liked" by the chair of the Danish Medical Association, Andreas Rudkjøbing.

The Danish Cancer Society's director, Leif Vestergaard, tweeted: "unacceptable confusion. And they always criticize others for conflicts of interest!"[119] What's the problem? I assume Vestergaard uses the Danish Cancer Society's letterhead when he writes letters related to his work.

The Danish Cancer Society's former chairman, Frede Olesen, tweeted: "A must read in Nature about HPV. Should be quoted in all Danish periodicals and newspapers and read by HPV sceptics or those who still have confidence in the Nordic Cochrane Centre."[120] He also wrote on Facebook: "Article in 'Nature,' the world's best scientific journal–clearly refutes the fear of the HPV vaccine and clearly denounces the dissemination of false science through the Nordic Cochrane Centre." This was pure fabrication. The article was not about our dissemination of science, the journal is not *Nature*, and we have never disseminated false science.

Journalist Ole Toft tweeted: "The Nordic Cochrane Centre (again) received harsh criticism—now in the HPV case in *Nature*. Both scientifically and by abusing Cochrane's credibility."[121] Again, pure fabrication, and there was no criticism of our scientific work in the e-letter.

Professor of psychiatry, Poul Videbech, on Facebook: "The Nordic Cochrane Centre gets criticism again—supported by the international Cochrane Collaboration Steering Group. This time in *Nature* itself . . . It is extremely worrying—is the Nordic Cochrane Centre closing down itself? What a tragedy for the Cochrane work!"[122] Once again, pure fabrication. We were not criticized by the Cochrane Steering Group.

Stinus Lindgren from a Danish political party upped the lies. On Facebook, he wrote that I had made comments against the HPV vaccine; that I had abused "Cochrane's good name and reputation"; and that "two of the leaders in Cochrane had asked the authors to publicly disclose this information to emphasize that this is not Cochrane's official view."[123] There was absolutely nothing about this in the letter from the Steering Group.

Line Emilie Fedders, the Danish Agency for Patient Safety: "Is the Nordic Cochrane Centre still on government finances with the aim of conducting impartial research?"[124]

It is inappropriate when people circulate derogatory and false comments about an issue they did not even investigate before they pressed the *send* button. I don't even think any of them had read the e-letter, as it is clear that it was not published in *Nature*. This "shoot before you ask" mentality not only undermines their authority, but also displays their hypocrisy: the authorities and similar institutions have complained wide and loud about fake news being spread on social media about dangers of vaccines while they happily contribute to spreading fake news themselves about a research group whose only interest it is to get as close to the truth as possible.

The editors of *NPJ Vaccines* also behaved inappropriately. We requested the opportunity to respond to the e-letter criticizing us, which was granted, but after exchange of many emails discussing nitty-gritty things in our reply, our reply had still not been published, more than two and a half years later, even though we had accommodated all the editors' wishes in November 2018.

Cochrane Review of the HPV Vaccines Was Flawed and Incomplete

A Cochrane review of the HPV vaccines was published on May 9, 2018.[125] It was long-awaited because of the controversy about the vaccines, but it was flawed and incomplete, and Cochrane rules for conflicts of interest were violated.

The gestation period was long, as the protocol for the review was already published seven years earlier.[126] Another curiosity is that the protocol had 14 authors, whereas the review had only 4. The history behind this change is not good PR for Cochrane.

Cochrane reviews must be independent of conflicts of interest associated with commercial sponsorship and should be conducted by people or organizations that are free of such bias,[127] but this is not always the case.

People employed by a company that has a real or potential financial interest in the outcome of the reviews are prohibited from being authors of Cochrane reviews,[128] but otherwise, they can be authors. This is problematic. A conflict of interest might be under way, and the employee might wish to conceal this, which would be similar to insider trading. Furthermore, having industry authors on Cochrane reviews decreases public trust in the reviews.

Another problem is that people can become authors even if in the last three years they have received financial support from sources that have a financial interest in the outcome. "In such cases, at the funding arbiter's discretion, and only where a majority of the review authors and lead author have no relevant COIs [conflicts of interest]," it may be possible for such people to be Cochrane authors.[129]

As I have argued elsewhere,[130] allowing almost half of the authors to receive financial support from the company whose product is being reviewed at a funding arbiter's discretion does not boost people's confidence in Cochrane's motto, "trusted evidence." It involves judgment and could lead to arbitrary, inconsistent, and disputable decisions. Furthermore, one or two people often dominate group work, and if these are conflicted, the process can go wrong. A funding arbiter is not likely to know anything about such concrete group dynamics.

The Cochrane editors turned a blind eye to the fact that far more than the allowed 50% of the authors on the protocol for the HPV vaccine review had major conflicts of interest in relation to the HPV vaccine manufacturers,[131] but many of them were removed after outsiders had protested.[132]

The lead and primary author of the Cochrane review, Marc Arbyn, had several financial ties to the vaccine manufacturers, which he failed to declare.[133] As this is not allowed according to Cochrane rules, my research group on the HPV vaccines complained about it. Our criticism was deferred to the Cochrane funding arbiters, which led to this amusing comment by a journalist in the *BMJ*: "asking them to arbitrate may not be seen as a perfect answer, given that the original declaration of interests in the HPV review said that its authors had been approved by the same committee, 'based on stringent Cochrane conflict of interest guidelines.'"[134]

The funding arbiters resolved that Arbyn had not breached the policy by not declaring his involvement in two organizations funded in whole or part by manufacturers of the vaccines and HPV tests because he had not gained personal financial benefit and because the support was provided through institutions.[135] Tom Jefferson from my research team pointed out that "the cash comes from sponsors even if it is routed through the North Pole [Santa Claus] and Mother Teresa of Calcutta."[136]

We published a criticism of the Cochrane review in July 2018.[137] We pointed out that the Cochrane review had missed nearly half of the eligible trials and was influenced by reporting bias and biased trial designs.

All 26 trials included in the Cochrane review used active comparators, either aluminium adjuvants or hepatitis vaccines. However, at a meeting in 2014, FDA acknowledged that this was not appropriate and suggested comparisons were adjuvanted vaccine vs. saline placebo and vs. unadjuvanted antigen.[138] FDA also suggested that there should be specific inquiries regarding symptoms consistent with autoimmune and neuroinflammatory diseases, with long postvaccination follow-up. It is astounding that FDA approved Gardasil even though none of these prerequisites were fulfilled.

We pointed out that GlaxoSmithKline had stated that its aluminium-based comparator causes harms: "higher incidences of myalgia might namely be attributable to the higher content of aluminium in the HPV vaccine (450 µg Al[OH]$_3$) than the content of aluminium in the HAV [hepatitis A] vaccine (225 µg Al[OH]$_3$)."[139] (The µg likely refers only to the aluminium content.)

The Cochrane authors mistakenly used the term placebo to describe the active comparators. They acknowledged that the assessment of adverse events was compromised by the use of adjuvants and hepatitis vaccines in the control group, but this statement can easily be missed, as it comes after 7,500 words about other issues in the discussion section under the heading "Potential biases in the review process," although it is not a bias in the review process, but in the design of the trials.

It is noteworthy that many girls and women were excluded from some of the large trials if they had received the adjuvants before or had a history of immunological or nervous system disorders.[140] These exclusion criteria lower the external validity of the trials, and they suggest that the vaccine manufacturers were worried about harms caused by the adjuvants. As such criteria are not listed as warnings on the package inserts, there could be more vaccine-related harms in clinical practice than in the trials.

In line with WHO recommendations, the Cochrane review used composite surrogate outcomes of various combinations of cell changes. The trials did not reflect clinical practice, however, as cervical screening often took place every six months, whereas in clinical practice, it is every three to five years. The Cochrane review did not describe any cancers, although two cervical cancers were reported on clinicaltrials.gov to have occurred in the vaccinated group in one of the trials.

The Cochrane authors concluded with "high certainty" that the risk of serious adverse events was similar in the HPV vaccine groups and the comparator groups. However, they overlooked several adverse events and failed to mention that several of the included trials did not report serious adverse events for the whole trial period, e.g., three Gardasil trials with a total of 21,441 girls or women with up to four years follow-up only reported serious adverse events occurring within 14 days postvaccination.

The Cochrane authors found more deaths in the HPV vaccine groups than in the comparator groups. The death rate was significantly increased in women above age 25, risk ratio 2.36 (1.10 to 5.03). The Cochrane authors considered that this was a chance occurrence since there was no pattern in the causes of death or in the time between vaccine administration and death. However, a death may be coded in a way that does not raise suspicion that the vaccine caused it. For example, *traumatic head injury* or *drowning* could have been caused by a syncope or near syncope, which is a recognized harm.

The Cochrane authors "planned requesting data from data owners, to fill in gaps with available unpublished data," but "due to constraints in time and other resources" they were unable to do so. Considering that seven years passed from the publication of the protocol to the review, lack of time seems a poor excuse for doing work of poor quality.

The Cochrane authors referred to many observational studies in their discussion that found no signals of harms associated with the HPV vaccines, but there were glaring omissions. They cited WHO's Global Advisory Committee on Vaccine Safety, which expressed "concerns about unjustified claims of harms," but not the study I have mentioned earlier, published online in September 2016 by the Uppsala Monitoring Centre, that found serious harms following HPV vaccination and evidence of underreporting.[141]

The Cochrane authors did not investigate whether the included trial data reported cases of POTS, CRPS, or other safety signals. Instead, they cited EMA that dismissed any causal relationship between POTS or CRPS and the vaccines, which is the same as saying that the Cochrane authors trusted the vaccine manufacturers, who we all know cannot be trusted. What a disgrace this is for Cochrane.

The Cochrane authors assessed the impact of industry funding and did not find significant effects. They stated that all trials but one were funded by the manufacturers. That is an inadequate basis on which to do a regression analysis (an analysis of trend). Moreover, that lone trial was sponsored by GlaxoSmithKline, which renders their analysis even more meaningless.[142]

Cochrane's PR was also highly suspect. It looked like a drug company announcing its new blockbuster. Six experts were cited on Cochrane's home-page, all from the United Kingdom, although Cochrane is an international organization. Two had financial conflicts of interest with the HPV vaccine manufacturers; a third was responsible for vaccinations in Public Health England, which promotes the HPV vaccines. None of the experts criticized the Cochrane review, which was highly praised for its rigor.

I felt it would be appropriate to change Cochrane's motto, *trusted evidence,* into *touted nonevidence,* or, as Tom Jefferson phrased it, garbage in, garbage out, with a nice little Cochrane logo on it.[143]

The Cochrane Empire Strikes Back

One would have thought it impossible to argue against us after we had pointed all this out,[144] but Cochrane headquarters tried. They had their brand to protect, which Cochrane CEO, Mark Wilson, who is a journalist, talks about incessantly while caring less about whether Cochrane gets the science right.[145]

Only a week after we published our peer-reviewed scientific critique of the Cochrane review, alerting the public that many studies and patients were missing and that the harms of the vaccines had been underestimated, we were heavily attacked by Cochrane's editor-in-chief and his deputy, who published a 30-page comment on the Cochrane website.[146] They claimed that we had substantially overstated our criticisms and concluded that we "made allegations that are not warranted and provided an inaccurate and sensationalized report. . . . We believe that there are questions to be asked about the rigour of the peer review and editorial review by *BMJ Evidence-Based Medicine*" (where we had published our criticism).

This illustrates a huge problem in the Cochrane leadership. The authors of the review did not respond to us, which is the appropriate thing to do. Instead, Cochrane used its nominal authority, which is an effective strategy for denigrating your opponents. In his book, *The Art of Always Being Right*, philosopher Arthur Schopenhauer calls it "Appeal to authority rather than reason."[147]

Cochrane reviews are based on the best available evidence, which we call evidence-based medicine (EBM), but this was "eminence-based medicine," which we all otherwise abhor.

People shun uncertainty and prefer definitive answers even when there are none. All over the world, the Cochrane editors' criticism of us has been interpreted as "the final word" in the debate. However, they did not address our most important concerns, and they thanked the first author of the HPV vaccine review and the coordinating editor of the Cochrane group that published the review for contributing to their report. If the editors had been interested in getting the science right, they would have offered us the same opportunity to comment, but it was not a scientific discussion or diplomacy; it was warfare, protecting the Cochrane flag.

Our criticism of the Cochrane HPV vaccine review is highly warranted. After we had done further detective work, we published an even stronger criticism, on September 17, 2018.[148] The Cochrane review should have included at least 35% (over 25,000) additional eligible females in its meta-analyses. Understandably, the Cochrane editors' unfounded allegations about poor editorial work at the journal where we published our initial critique upset its editors, who asked the Cochrane editors to be concrete and invited them to publish their response in the journal. This they didn't do, and they would have lost the battle.

We demonstrated that the two Cochrane silverbacks ignored our criticism of incomplete reporting of serious adverse events, were inaccurate in the description of the active controls, did not consider the substantial bias caused by use of surrogate outcomes, incompletely assessed the authors' conflicts of interest and ignored additional ones, did not acknowledge that media coverage should be balanced and free from financial conflicts of interest, appeared to advocate scientific censorship, and substantially ignored several of our criticisms and important evidence of bias.

* * *

Even deaths were misreported in the Cochrane review, and there were many other problems that could have been avoided if the Cochrane authors had looked carefully in the journal publications they used or in the freely available clinical study reports on GlaxoSmithKline's trial register that they assessed.

The HPV vaccines are expensive blockbusters generating billions of dollars of revenue, and the Cochrane review ought to have been totally independent of any financial conflicts of interest. The Cochrane editors-in-chief are confident that the Cochrane authors have no relevant conflicts of interest, but we gave many examples of such conflicts.[149] For example, in 2018, the Cochrane review's first author, Marc Arbyn, was on the EUROGIN program committee where Merck is a platinum sponsor, and the last author was sponsored by Merck via Medscape.[150]

As noted, the Cochrane editors-in-chief seem to advocate scientific censorship. They wrote that:

> Scientific debate is to be welcomed, and differences of opinion between different Cochrane "voices" is not unexpected. However, public confidence may be undermined, unnecessary anxiety caused, and public health put at risk if that debate is not undertaken in an appropriate way. This is especially true when such debates take place in public. There is already a formidable and growing anti-vaccination lobby. If the result of this controversy is reduced uptake of the vaccine among young women, this has the potential to lead to women suffering and dying unnecessarily from cervical cancer.[151]

We believe our criticism of the Cochrane HPV review is justified and has general interest, and that debates over sources of evidence must take place in public, especially when public health interventions are at stake.

But that is not how the Cochrane leadership sees it. There is no doubt that my criticism of the Cochrane HPV vaccine review played a major role in my expulsion from Cochrane.[152] It is not surprising that editors of some of our most prestigious medical journals see the Cochrane editors' reaction toward us as a symptom of Cochrane's moral downfall and that there were articles in *Science, Nature, BMJ, Lancet,* and elsewhere about my unjustified expulsion from Cochrane.[153]

Our criticism of the Cochrane review is based on evidence we had studied very carefully for over two years. My research group has worked with the clinical study reports we obtained from EMA about the HPV vaccine trials, and we therefore have a unique knowledge about these trials. The clinical study reports can take up thousands of pages for just one trial, and they are far more reliable than the short reports the drug companies publish in medical journals, particularly in relation to harms. We are likely the only ones in the world who have read 60,000 pages of study reports.

Many people have criticized that, in 2016, the Cochrane Collaboration received a grant of $1.15 million from the Bill and Melinda Gates Foundation, as one of Gates' major projects seems to be propagating the use of the HPV vaccines throughout the world.[154] We can only speculate if Cochrane's actions were driven by fear of losing future financial support from the Gates foundation.

Our Systematic Review of the HPV Vaccine Trials

Our systematic review of the HPV vaccine trials[155] is much more reliable than the Cochrane review, as we based it on clinical study reports and not on publications. It was published as part of a PhD thesis on March 12, 2019,[156] and accepted for publication in *Systematic Reviews*, a journal owned by Springer, on March 6, 2019.[157] However, a year later, it had still not been published, although the journal promises publication within 20 days of acceptance. Our email correspondence took up an astonishing 66 pages, and we had been given a total of 20 apologies and a variety of odd, contradictory, and implausible reasons for why our paper had not yet been published. During that year, *Systematic Reviews* had published 309 papers. On February 16, 2020, we wrote to Springer that it seemed they deliberately delayed the publication and highlighted that:

> If this is the case, it is scientific censorship that borders on scientific misconduct and fraud. We have a big network with renowned scientists, many connections with the international media, and a strong social media presence. If *Springer Nature*, *BMC*, and *Systematic Reviews* fail to publish our papers before 1 March 2020, we are obliged to alarm our fellow scientists and the international and social media about *Springer Nature's*, *BMC's* and *Systemic Reviews'* editorial practices. We will also involve the Nordic Cochrane Centre's and the Danish taxpayers' legal teams if the 1 March 2020 deadline is not met.

This caused Springer to publish our review with record speed, on February 28, 2020.[158]

EMA released its study reports to us with extraordinary slowness. After three years, we went ahead with what we had, which was the major trials.[159] The 24 clinical study reports we included comprised 79% of the total eligible sample of participants.[160]

Against all odds, as active comparators were used in the control groups, we found that the HPV vaccines increased serious nervous system disorders significantly: 72 vs. 46 patients, risk ratio 1.49 (1.02 to 2.16; p = 0.04), number needed to harm (NNH, the number vaccinated per one person harmed) 1,325.[161] We called this an exploratory analysis, but it is the most important of our analyses because the suspected harms to the autonomic nervous system were what caused EMA to assess vaccine safety in 2015.

POTS and CRPS are rare syndromes that are difficult to identify, and we knew that the companies had deliberately concealed what they found. This was also illustrated by the fact that not a single case of POTS or CRPS was mentioned in the clinical study reports. To assess whether there were signs and symptoms consistent with POTS or CRPS in the data, we did another exploratory analysis where we asked a blinded physician (Louise Brinth) with clinical expertise in POTS and CRPS to assess the reported MedDRA preferred terms (which are code terms the companies use to categorize and report adverse events) as definitely, probably, probably not, or definitely not associated with the syndromes. As an example, Brinth judged the MedDRA terms *dizziness postural* and *pain in extremity* to be definitely associated with POTS and CRPS, respectively. Brinth was blinded to the allocation groups and outcome data.

The HPV vaccines significantly increased serious harms that were judged definitely associated with POTS or CRPS: for POTS, 56 vs. 26, risk ratio 1.92 (1.21 to 3.07), NNH 1,073, p = 0.006; and for CRPS, 95 vs. 57, risk ratio 1.54 (1.11 to 2.14), NNH 906, p = 0.01. New onset diseases that were judged definitely associated with POTS were also increased: 3,675 vs. 3,352, risk ratio 1.08 (1.01 to 1.15), NNH 144, p = 0.03. The significance of tests should be interpreted with caution, however, as a participant might have been included more than once in the analysis.

We communicated these results for the first time at the Nordic Cochrane Centre's 25th Anniversary Research Symposium on October 12, 2018, and again in March 2019 and February 2020.[162]

Public Reactions to Our Findings of Harm

The media were present at our anniversary symposium but did not pay attention to our findings that our PhD student, Lars Jørgensen, presented.

When he defended his thesis half a year later, the media announced that there was nothing to worry about and that I had chosen three examiners who were all biased against the HPV vaccines. The headline in a major

Danish newspaper was: "The University of Copenhagen approves controversial HPV research: 'Is it about promoting some anti-vaccine agenda?'"
[163] It was like religious intolerance, following the well-known confession for vaccines, "are you for or against," that the three examiners were described as vaccine heretics, which they are not. And the research was not at all controversial; it was of high quality. The university rejected this primitivism: "We have considered that the examiners' competencies are adequate. We sustain academic freedom in research and therefore do not consider people's attitudes." The university would have rejected my proposed examiners if they had been conflicted. One was Rebecca Chandler from the Uppsala Monitoring Centre, who knows a lot about the HPV vaccines and has been EMA's rapporteur for one of them. Another was Kim Varming, an immunologist with an interest in the vaccines and an expert on harms caused by autoimmune reactions. The third, John Brodersen, led the defense. This person must be employed by the university in a senior position, which limits the choices, but he has a long-standing interest in cancer screening and works at the Department for General Practice, which I found ideal.

In March 2015, three months before EMA started assessing the harms of the HPV vaccines, TV2, one of the two major TV channels in Denmark, showed a documentary about harms that some girls had experienced after the vaccination.[164] The announcement of the program said that about 1,000, or one per 500 girls vaccinated, had reported side effects of the vaccine to the National Board of Health, 283 of which were serious. The documentary was very good, and it stated that no one knew with certainty whether the symptoms were caused by the vaccine. Nonetheless, a storm of protests was raised against the TV channel from the authorities and organizations with special interests like the Danish Cancer Society, which had the result that the editors do not dare touch this subject again.

The program had a dramatic effect. Although the vaccine is free, coverage dropped from 90% to just 25% in two years.[165] A spokesperson from the National Board of Health warned that this could cause deaths, but the board was criticized for not listening. A master in public health had experienced that the Danish Cancer Society had censored her on its Facebook page, where she had criticized the vaccine so that she could no longer upload comments. It did not strengthen the credibility of the authorities when TV2 via the Freedom of Information Act discovered that the National Board of Health had failed to communicate warnings about the vaccine.

The board acknowledged that it had been misleading when they declared that the vaccine was safe and added that they needed to articulate more sympathy and commitment. There had already been a series of critical newspaper articles about the vaccine in 2013, and the 2015 TV documentary's main focus was that the girls felt the system had treated them badly.

The National Board of Health reacted with considerable arrogance all the time. On its website, the board provided a list of references in support of its position, but—just like in the Cochrane review of the HPV vaccines—there was a glaring omission: the important study carried out by the Uppsala Monitoring Centre appeared nowhere.[166]

The board's director, Søren Brostrøm, talked about alternative facts when researchers were skeptical of the work done by the drug companies and EMA. He launched the idea that people are opposed to the HPV vaccine because we live in "a postfactual society."[167] Denigrating remarks like these can have the opposite effect of the intended one.

At a meeting of the Danish Medical Association in August 2017, I informed the participants about EMA's poor work and that placebo-controlled trials had not been carried out. Brostrøm became very aggressive and alleged that there was a trial where 4,000 had received placebo and that I had climbed high up in a tree and could be mistaken. I responded that I didn't climb trees but had both feet on the ground, since, in contrast to him, I hadn't claimed anything about the safety or harms of the vaccines.

Six months later, in a newspaper article that was an attempt at character assassination of me,[168] Brostrøm said I was looking for a tiny hair in the medical soup instead of looking at the soup, and he criticized that I had used my energy on complaining about EMA.

The official handling of the HPV vaccine controversy—pretending we have sufficient knowledge when we don't—has caused many people to lose confidence in the authorities. In Japan, where an unusually high rate of harms has been reported, vaccination is no longer recommended by the authorities, and the vaccination rate has decreased from 80% to less than 1%[169]

Vaccine coverage in Denmark has gone up, but in many areas, it was low for a long time. The low vaccination rate was described by the Board of Health as a catastrophe lurking just around the corner if we do not get that rate up. It is difficult to see any lurking catastrophe, which I shall discuss in the next section. Perhaps it is more of a lurking catastrophe for Brostrøm. Several directors for the National Board of Health have been fired in the past when they did not live up to political expectations.

Should Girls Get Vaccinated?

The alternative to reducing the risk of getting cervical cancer by vaccination is to attend screening. Screening is highly effective and can find cell changes that can be removed long before they develop into cancer many years later.

Since the HPV vaccine only provides partial protection, it is recommended to go to screening even if you are vaccinated. It may therefore seem irrational to get vaccinated, but that is not the case. Due to the frequency of detected cell changes, screening leads to many conizations (removal of part of the cervix). Conization can lead to severe bleeding, and it doubles the risk of preterm birth, from about 5% to 11%.[170] This is a significant harm, but it can be reduced. Many cell changes never develop into cancer, and most disappear again.[171] It is therefore possible to adopt a wait-and-see approach, with regular cervical smears, which may substantially reduce conizations.[172]

Studies suggest that the vaccine protects more broadly than for the targeted HPV types. In Scotland, bivalent vaccination against types 16 and 18 led to an 86% decrease in cervical intraepithelial neoplasia grade 3 (which is not cancer; it is only cell changes, also called stage 0 carcinoma in situ) and to some herd protection.[173] A systematic review found that the prevalence of HPV 16 and 18 decreased by 83% among young girls, and of HPV 31, 33, and 45 by 54%.[174] Anogenital warts decreased by 67% among girls and 48% among boys.

The HPV vaccine controversy is a typical example of the clash between public health and individual health, which we also saw for the influenza vaccines. The public health perspective is that cervical cancer is a terrible disease; that we can avoid many deaths through vaccination; that the harms are trivial compared to the benefits; and that everyone in a given age range should get vaccinated. But as citizens, we should always ask: What's in it for me? Dying from cervical cancer is very rare. Only some 100 people in Denmark die every year, whereas about 14,000, both sexes included, die from smoking. Thus, we would accomplish far more if we used resources for preventing young people from starting smoking rather than convincing their parents that their daughters and sons should get vaccinated against HPV.

A key issue is that we don't know what the effect is. The vaccines lower the risk of infection with some HPV strains that are known to cause cancer and the risk of cell changes, but they are only about 70% protective against the targeted HPV strains, and other strains can cause cancer. We don't know if these other strains will take over, or for how many years the vaccines are protective, but we do know that viruses mutate. It is very likely that the vaccines will reduce deaths from cervical cancer, but it has not been documented.

Another key issue is when the expected benefit will come. The propaganda focuses on young girls with cervical cancer, but about half of those who die from cervical cancer are over 70 years of age. Only about 12 women in Denmark under 45 years of age die of cervical cancer each year. If we assume that all 12-year-old girls become vaccinated and that the vaccine is 70% effective, then about 8 women will be spared each year.

In Denmark, around 32,000 girls are 12 years old. Assuming we can save 8 of them each year, the number needed to vaccinate to save one is 4,000, which is a very small benefit. We don't even know if this estimate is correct. If the extensive propaganda lulls women into believing they are safe and no longer need to attend screening, there will be more cases of cancer than predicted.

A third key issue is that we don't know the number needed to vaccinate to seriously harm one person. We cannot deduce this number from the randomized trials, not only because of the lack of placebo controls, but also because the drug companies have actively tried to avoid registering any harms. Some of the doctors have been complicit in this, and some have suggested that these girls merely suffer from psychological problems. That may be the case sometimes, but postulating that all of them are having such issues is not only wrong, but insulting.

A review of the published trials from 2017 found more deaths in the vaccine groups than in the control groups (14 vs. 3, p = 0.01).[175] The review also mentioned a large trial that compared 9-valent Gardasil with Gardasil in 14,215 women.[176] In this trial, there were far more serious local reactions with the 9-valent vaccine (e.g., 272 vs. 109 cases of swelling). A supplementary appendix revealed that there were also more serious systemic adverse events in girls receiving the 9-valent vaccine than in those receiving the 4-valent vaccine (3.3% vs. 2.6%, p = 0.01).[177] The number needed to harm was only 141,[178] and it would undoubtedly have been even smaller if the control group had not received Gardasil, too.

This result suggests that, contrary to EMA's reassuring messages, adjuvants are harmful, not only locally, but also systemically. Gardasil 9 contains 500 µg of aluminium, i.e. more of the AAHS adjuvant than Gardasil that contains only 225 µg.[179] Yet only 4 of the 416 serious adverse events were judged to be vaccine-related by the trial authors.[180] It is "interesting" when clinical investigators—many of whom had many conflicts of interest with vaccine manufacturers—decide that only 1% of the serious adverse events are vaccine-related. Where did they publish this? In *New England Journal of Medicine*, of course, which one of my colleagues has dubbed *New England Journal of Medicalization*. And how could they make such a decision when both groups received Gardasil? It just cannot be done.

As of May 2018, WHO's pharmacovigilance database, VigiBase, managed by the Uppsala Monitoring Centre, contained 499 deaths reported as related to HPV vaccination.[181] It is difficult to know which of these deaths were caused by the vaccine and which were coincidental, but sometimes there is little doubt that the vaccine was the cause.

In Spain, a young woman with asthma had a severe exacerbation when she received the first shot of the vaccine. Despite that, she got a second shot a month later and developed severe dyspnea and seizures 12 hours later. She was admitted to an intensive care unit, where she died two weeks later. The judicial ruling acknowledged a causal link to the vaccine.[182]

In Sweden, a girl drowned in a bathtub after the vaccination. According to information I received from the Uppsala Monitoring Centre, the girl developed symptoms within two weeks of her first vaccination and had a clinical course dominated by headache, fatigue, and syncope spells. She was referred to a pediatric neurologist, who diagnosed her with "epilepsy" based upon some mild EEG changes. It seems more likely that she drowned because of fainting than because of "epilepsy."[183]

No one in a leading official position wants to see the harms. In 2013, WHO introduced new criteria for the assessment of causality of individual adverse events following vaccination.[184] They make it almost impossible to detect signals of serious harm—including deaths—after vaccinations.[185] I have never seen so many critical comments on PubMed as those related to the abstract about the new WHO criteria. Both papers make for chilling reading.[186]

As noted above, the heavy propaganda about the safety of HPV vaccines has had the effect that many doctors do not report their suspicions of serious harms. They know they could get in trouble.

In September 2008, when the immunization program for Cervarix had just started, Kent Woods, head of the UK drug agency, sent a letter to doctors asking them to report any suspected adverse reactions. One year later, Woods sent a second letter mentioning that there had been newspaper stories about adverse events including chronic fatigue, but that—based upon reported events against expected background rates—there was no reason to believe a causal link existed. Since the doctors were now told that their reporting had not identified problems, the second letter probably discouraged some of them from reporting not only chronic fatigue, but also symptoms of POTS and CRPS. The letter was sent right in the middle of the study period of an investigation that was used by EMA in November 2015 to dismiss concerns about serious neurological harms of the HPV vaccines.[187] All authors of the paper reporting on this investigation were employees at the UK drug agency, and their paper did not mention Woods's second letter.

Nonetheless, despite all the reassurances about the safety of the HPV vaccines, the number of spontaneously reported adverse reactions to the UK drug regulator in a 10-year period ending in April 2015 exceeded by far those for any other vaccine or combination of vaccines.[188]

There have, of course, been a number of observational studies in reaction to the suspicion of harms, but—in contrast to the best studies of the measles vaccine that rejected the hypothesis that it causes autism—they have not been convincing. When serious harms are very rare, and very difficult to diagnose, and when both drug companies and the authorities contribute to underreporting by assuring us there is nothing to worry about, they can easily be overlooked in such studies.

There are surprisingly few studies. A PubMed search on *hpv vaccine pots* in June 2019 yielded only 27 records, none of which described studies that had compared vaccinated with unvaccinated females.

The review of the published trials from 2017[189] I mentioned just above was vitriolically attacked on a Danish science site,[190] which is supposed to be neutral but publishes quite positive articles about the HPV vaccines. It was even postulated that the review came very close to scientific misconduct. In my view, the criticism lacked merit, and it was more a question of the critics not liking what the researchers had found and wanting to protect the vaccines.

The authors had reviewed not only the randomized trials, but also postmarketing adverse events case series, and they were criticized for not having included three studies. This criticism was inappropriate. Using the authors' search strategy (*HPV vaccine* and diagnoses that have been associated to HPV vaccination: complex regional pain syndrome, fibromyalgia, chronic fatigue syndrome, postural orthostatic tachycardia syndrome, or ovarian failure), I also failed to find the three studies on PubMed. But since the critics believed they are important, I shall discuss them.

One study included almost 4 million females in Denmark and Sweden, around 800,000 of whom were vaccinated.[191] It did not find an increased risk of multiple sclerosis or of other demyelinating diseases. Not terribly interesting, as these diseases are not among the "prime suspects."

A Danish study found that 316 vaccinated females had increased care seeking in the two years before receiving the first HPV vaccine compared to 163,910 controls.[192] The authors concluded that prevaccination morbidity should be taken into account in the evaluation of vaccine safety signals. This is prudent advice, but I have two reservations. All the increases were small, between 1.5 and 2 times, and the lower end of the confidence intervals was close to one, which, in observational studies, means that these differences could easily have been caused by confounding (those who complain about health problems may also be those who tend to get vaccinated). Further, even if true, these results were not unexpected. Brinth found that many of the girls with POTS were elite sportswomen, and such people would be expected to consult doctors more often than others for injuries and diseases of the digestive system or the musculoskeletal system, get physiotherapy more often, and go to a psychologist/psychiatrist more often. It is well known, for example, that competitive swimming is highly demanding and leads to increases in exactly those variables the researchers reported on.

In the third study, the researchers had included 70,265 Swedish females (16% of whom were vaccinated) with at least one of 49 prespecified autoimmune diseases, and they looked for new-onset autoimmune disease within 180 days of vaccination.[193] They found a slightly reduced risk of new diseases, incidence rate ratio 0.77 (0.65 to 0.93), which is reassuring but unconvincing, as the upper end of the confidence interval was close to one.

Such studies cannot remove the suspicion that the HPV vaccine causes serious neurological harms and other serious harms in susceptible people. We need focused research where we study the affected females rather than large epidemiological studies, which cannot give us the answer. A classic example is Guillain-Barré syndrome and tetanus vaccination.[194] Despite multiple observational studies showing no increased risk of the syndrome at the population level, there is a famous case report of a 42-year-old man who received tetanus toxoid on three occasions over 13 years and developed a self-limited episode of Guillain-Barré each time.

As already noted, the symptoms of dysautonomia are so diffuse that they are often overlooked, not only by the clinicians but also by researchers studying databases of reported adverse events. In the United States, for example, researchers reviewed POTS reports submitted to the Vaccine Adverse Event Reporting System (VAERS).[195] They searched for reports of POTS following HPV vaccination from 2006 to 2015. There was a huge amount of VAERS reports following HPV vaccination, 40,735, but they found only 29 POTS reports that "fully met diagnostic criteria."

In Denmark, 26 cases of POTS were registered after vaccination, about the same as in the United States, although this country has 60 times as many inhabitants as Denmark. Since the Danish cases have been carefully assessed, the US numbers are hugely unreliable and speak volumes about how unreliable observational studies in this area are.

All the US researchers were employed by the CDC or the FDA—agencies that are not interested in finding harms of vaccines. They should perhaps have looked harder in the VAERS database.

In another study, published in 2009, only three years after approval of Gardasil in the United States, researchers from the CDC reported that the most frequently reported adverse event to VAERS was syncope, with 8.2 reports per 100,000 doses; the next two were 7.5 for local site reactions and 6.8 for dizziness.[196] Ninety percent of the syncopes occurred on the same day of the vaccination, and there were 200 falls that resulted in head injuries.

The authorities should have paid attention to the harms of the vaccinations, instead of ignoring them, as EMA did. The signals of possible harm have primarily come from three countries: spontaneous reports of complex regional pain syndrome (CRPS) in Japan,[197] POTS in Denmark,[198] and long-lasting fatigue in the Netherlands.[199]

EMA stated in 2015 that the "benefits of HPV vaccines continue to outweigh their risks."[200] There are four problems with this statement: we don't know what the benefits are; it is not just *theoretical risks*, it is *real harms*; we don't know enough about what the harms are; and it is subjective to compare benefits and harms, as they are different. Only if they are the same, e.g., deaths, can we compare them objectively and indisputably.

As noted, my wife is a professor of clinical microbiology. Both of us got all the recommended childhood vaccinations and also gave them to our two daughters. We had not perceived vaccines to be a problem before the HPV vaccine was offered to our oldest daughter in 2008. Already back then, there were debates about rare but serious harms possibly caused by the vaccine, and we were in doubt. We vaccinated both of our girls, but today, after my own research on this vaccine, we would not have done it. There are too many uncertainties, and screening is a highly effective alternative.

What we need are large randomized trials conducted independently of the drug industry. Such trials could compare different vaccines, and vaccines versus nothing or a saline placebo, and harms could be carefully monitored, with objective tests such as the head-up tilt test for POTS where the patient's blood pressure, pulse, and condition are monitored when rising from a lying position.

Should Boys Get Vaccinated?

The top entry in a Google search on *hpv vaccination of boys* is information from the CDC. Not a trustworthy source, but let's see what the argument is.[201]

Headline: "Every year in the United States, over 13,000 men get cancers caused by human papillomavirus (HPV). HPV vaccination could prevent most of these cancers from ever developing."

Scaring people by big numbers is the archetype of health propaganda. How many males die from these cancers, and at what age? There is no information about this.

The website goes on: "HPV infections can cause cancers of the back of the throat (oropharyngeal cancer), anus, and penis in men. Cancers of the back of the throat have surpassed cervical cancer as the most common type of cancer caused by HPV. Unlike cervical cancer in women, there are no recommended screening tests." Okay, I got it. Worse than cervical cancer. Surely all boys must be vaccinated. But, oops! Using that kind of argument, it is smoking we should primarily prevent, not HPV infection.

"Take advantage of any medical visit—such as an annual health checkup or physicals for sports, camp or college—to ask the doctor about what shots your preteens and teens need."

Oh no! The United States is frightening when it comes to healthcare. Wake up! Our review of all the randomized trials showed that annual health checks don't work and are likely harmful.[202] And why on Earth have physicals before sports, camp, or college? So, don't "ask your doctor" to have these and refuse if your doctor suggests them.

"HPV vaccination provides safe, effective, and long-lasting protection against HPV cancers." Really? Do we know if HPV vaccination provides safe and effective protection against HPV cancers in boys or homosexual men? No, we don't. The CDC link to safety only mentions the effect in females.

Let's look up the annual number of cancer deaths in males. In the United States, deaths due to cancers in the throat, anus, or penis (or surrounding tissues) were 1% of the total cancer deaths.[203] If the HPV vaccine offers 70% protection, it means that 0.7% of all cancer deaths in males can be prevented by the vaccine.

It is not difficult to save many more male lives by spending public money more wisely than giving a huge amount to Merck and GlaxoSmithKline to vaccinate boys against HPV.

Japanese Encephalitis: A Worked-Through Example of Finding the Evidence

I have discussed in detail four vaccines that are often in the media, and which are very different in terms of whether we need them and whom we should believe.

At one end of the spectrum is the measles vaccine, which we should all have; the authorities are right in their recommendations; and parents and others who think it causes autism are wrong. At the other end is the influenza vaccine, which I believe we should not take, and the authorities, WHO included, have published a lot of seriously misleading information. In-between is the HPV vaccine, which is controversial. It is not necessary because screening for cervical cancer is highly effective; the authorities have been dishonest about the many uncertainties related to the vaccine and its adjuvant; and parents who have reported serious neurological harms have often been right. The coronavirus vaccines are also in-between, as children and some countries do not seem to need them, and as nothing is known about their long-term harms. Next, I shall give an example of how you can look up the evidence yourself instead of blindly trusting the authorities.

Travelers are offered many vaccines, but they are not all equally essential. We should try to find out where the balance is between the benefits and harms and when it tips in either direction. I have worked through this example earlier[1] but will expand on it here.

Imagine you find out the risk of getting infected during a two-week stay in a tropical country is about 1 in 1000. This can be a bit tricky to estimate because the risk may vary with the time of year, e.g., if the infection is transmitted by mosquitoes, and it can be increased during epidemics. If the risk of developing a serious complication to the disease is 1 in 50, it means that your risk of getting badly harmed without vaccination will be 1 in 50,000 (1000 x 50). If the vaccine package insert or other online information states that the risk of serious harm from the vaccination is 1 in 10,000, it means that you can travel to such places five times unvaccinated without exposing yourself to a greater risk of being seriously harmed than if you had been vaccinated.

This example is somewhat simplified. For example, the harms from the infection are not the same as those from the vaccine, unless we are only interested in the death risk with and without vaccination, in which case they are directly comparable.

* * *

Vaccination against Japanese encephalitis is sometimes recommended in guidelines, but what is the risk of becoming infected? When googling *japanese encephalitis*, various suggestions appear while typing, including *incidence*, which is the number of annual cases. The first link was to WHO and states that the annual incidence of clinical disease varies both across and within endemic countries (areas where the disease regularly occurs), ranging from less than 1 to more than 10 cases per 100,000 population or higher during outbreaks.[2] A literature review estimated that nearly 68,000 clinical cases globally occur each year, with a case-fatality rate of about 25%. The disease primarily affects children. Most adults in endemic countries have natural immunity after childhood infection.

If we use the high-risk estimate for getting infected, 10 per 100,000, which is 1 per 10,000, we get the risk in two weeks by dividing this risk by 26, which is 1 per 260,000.

Of those who survive, 20–30% will suffer permanent intellectual, behavioral, or neurological sequelae such as paralysis, recurrent seizures, or the inability to speak. There is no cure, but according to WHO, "safe and effective vaccines are available."[3] You should never believe such reassuring statements, which is industry jargon. Nothing is both safe and effective; effectiveness always comes with a price. You will need to find out how often people get seriously harmed with and without the vaccine, and what the harms are.

In healthcare, people rarely use the term "harms." They talk about side effects, which is a euphemism for the inevitable—some people will be harmed and in rare cases even die after having received a vaccine. As long as this tradition prevails, it is best to search for side effects. Adverse reactions, adverse events, adverse effects, and harms are also useful terms.

Nonetheless, I tried the harms option and googled *japanese encephalitis vaccine harms*. A report from 1996 noted that 54% of vaccinated persons reported one or more adverse effects, 2.2% of those reporting reactions (i.e., 1% of those vaccinated) sought medical advice, and 1.8% (1% of those vaccinated) were unfit for work for an average of 2.2 days.[4] The authors noted that the amount of systemic reactions might indicate a potential hazard of serious anaphylactic reactions and that Japanese encephalitis is an extremely rare disease in travelers.

Next—since serious harms are often downplayed or omitted (most entries I looked at were about common side effects)—I included *FDA* in my search. When I did this in 2017, the first entry was the product information for a vaccine sold by Sanofi Pasteur. It said that people should not embark on international travel within 10 days of the vaccination because of the possibility of delayed allergic reactions, and they should have ready access to medical care.

The information retrieved so far did not exactly describe a vaccine with trivial harms, but it becomes worse. Adverse reactions include immediate generalized urticaria (hives) or angioedema (giant hives), and such reactions could be delayed and involve the extremities, face, and oropharynx. Highly technical language, which patients do not understand (e.g., oropharynx is mouth and throat). They therefore do not understand how dangerous these reactions are, and that they could kill them through suffocation.

The product information also noted that the decision to administer the vaccine should balance the risks of exposure to the virus and for developing illness, the availability and acceptability of repellents and other protective measures, and the side effects of vaccination.

It is great to see this in a product information section. I am convinced Sanofi Pasteur did not get this idea themselves but were asked by FDA to include it because the agency was worried about vaccine safety.

Systemic side effects—principally fever, headache, malaise, rash, and other reactions, such as chills, dizziness, myalgia (muscle pain), nausea, vomiting, and abdominal pain—have been reported in approximately 10% of vaccinees. Very rarely, deaths have occurred with vaccine-associated encephalitis.

What a vaccine! What I miss in the package insert is information on the number of deaths caused by the vaccine. I also miss information that Japanese encephalitis is transmitted by mosquitoes, which means that bed nets and insect repellents offer good protection. Since the vaccine can be deadly, there must be situations where more people die from being vaccinated than from the infection if not vaccinated; this depends on the risk of getting infected and on how cautious you are with avoiding mosquitoes.

Sometimes we need to make decisions on an insufficient basis, which is the case here. In my view, most travelers to endemic areas should avoid being vaccinated. Although I have visited the tropics many times, I have never been vaccinated against Japanese encephalitis because I knew that the risk of infection was extremely low. WHO has reservations, too. It recommends travelers get vaccinated when spending extensive time in endemic areas.

Danish Handbook for Patients recommends vaccination of travelers who, for more than four weeks, travel to areas where the disease exists and when traveling for shorter durations during periods of outbreaks of the disease.

The CDC tells you to get the vaccine if recommended and to "Talk to your doctor about your travel plans: Your doctor can help you decide if you need the JE vaccine based on the length of your trip, the areas where you will be traveling, and your planned activities."[5]

The Danish recommendations mean that if you go on vacation to Thailand for a week, you should only get vaccinated if there is an outbreak of the disease. In the United States, your doctor will likely persuade you to get vaccinated in any case, for his or her own safety in order to avoid a lawsuit about malpractice should anything happen to you. The US recommendation is typical for America, where ads for drugs on TV always end with "Talk to your doctor." But in an area with so much uncertainly, it is unlikely your doctor will be qualified to advise you. It is more a matter of the authorities avoiding any responsibility by simply passing the buck. Just like doctors, organizations protect themselves by being overcautious because, if anybody dies, they can point to the fact that they did warn people.

I do not blame them. They are in a difficult position. But my conclusion is that we should look up the facts ourselves rather than blindly following official advice. As I do not want to be sued by wealthy American lawyers, I shall make it absolutely clear that I have not given you any advice about becoming vaccinated or not, I just worked through an example. The decision is entirely yours.

8

Childhood Vaccination Programs

These differ a lot from country to country, which reflects not only differences in wealth, but also widely different interpretations of the evidence and differences in political pressures and industry lobbying (which is often the same).

The Danish childhood vaccination program offers free vaccination against diphtheria, tetanus, pertussis (whooping cough), polio, Hib (Haemophilus influenzae type b), pneumococci, measles, mumps, rubella, and human papillomavirus (HPV) for girls aged 12 to 18 years.[1]

In the United States, the same 10 vaccinations are recommended, but there are 7 more: hepatitis B, rotavirus, influenza (annually), varicella, hepatitis A, meningococcal serogroup A, C, W, Y, and meningococcal serogroup B.[2]

In the United Kingdom, 15 vaccinations are recommended.[3] Compared with those in the United States, varicella and hepatitis A are not on the list.

Since the UK healthcare system in recent years has become more and more similar to that in the United States,[4] it is not surprising that routine recommendations of vaccines are also similar. The similarities are also obvious in regard to the poor returns of the money invested. The healthy life expectancy is lower in the United Kingdom than in most other European countries, and the prevalence of chronic disease and disability lies between that in the Unites States and the rest of Europe.[5] I do not suggest, of course, that the reasons for the poor health outcomes are due to more vaccinations. The main reasons are increased privatization, increased specialization of healthcare, and increased usage of screening tests, with subsequent overdiagnosis and overtreatment.[6]

Diphtheria, Tetanus, Polio, Pertussis, and Haemophilus Influenzae Type B

These vaccines are often given to infants in combinations that vary from country to country and from time to time, and even within the same country, according to the age of the child. There are trivalent vaccines (diphtheria, tetanus, and polio or pertussis), tetravalent (all four, for revaccination at age five), and pentavalent (all five, or other combinations). Apart from polio, these diseases are caused by bacteria.

None of the combination vaccines contain live attenuated microorganisms. As Aaby's studies have shown, we don't know what we are doing when we combine several vaccines (see Chapter 1). His research group found that live vaccines decrease total mortality, while nonlive vaccines increase total mortality; that the sequence of vaccinations also seems to be important for total mortality (ending with a live vaccine is best); and that the effect could be different in girls and boys.

These observations make it very difficult to choose the best options for childhood vaccinations because vaccination programs do not take into account Aaby's findings. In Denmark, it is recommended to give the pentavalent vaccine at age 3 months plus a pneumococcus vaccine, which contains polysaccharide from the bacterium, but this is not followed by vaccination with a live attenuated vaccine like measles. The six vaccines are given again after 5 and 12 months, and not before 15 months do children receive their first dose of the MMR vaccine (the measles, mumps, and rubella in the vaccine are all attenuated live viruses). Fortunately, at least one trial is currently ongoing where some children already get the MMR vaccine after 6 months and the others after 15 months.

Wikipedia is often a good starting point if you wish to study the issues yourself. About Haemophilus influenzae type b, for example, it states:[7]

> Prior to introduction of the conjugate vaccine, Hib was a leading cause of childhood meningitis, pneumonia, and epiglottitis (inflammation in the flap at the base of the tongue which can be lethal due to suffocation) in the United States, causing an estimated 20,000 cases a year in the early 1980s, mostly in children under 5 years old. Since routine vaccination began, the incidence of Hib disease has declined by more than 99%.

When you see data like this, choosing vaccination is the obvious choice.

The five diseases the pentavalent vaccine provides good protection against are so horrible that I believe our children should get the vaccine, but

Aaby's studies worry me (see a few lines down). I would prefer it be followed by one of the attenuated live vaccines, which raises the question of how early in life we dare give such vaccines to infants with a not yet sufficiently developed immune system. In Guinea-Bissau, BCG and the polio vaccine are given at birth and the measles vaccine at 4 months.

These issues need urgent testing in randomized trials that are large enough to study the effects of the vaccines on total mortality. Presently, no one can say for sure what would be the best thing to do. In such situations, my hunch is to accept the advice from the authorities. Although it is sometimes misleading, there is work behind it. Some people—hopefully not with conflicts of interest and hopefully not biased—have gone through at least some of the scientific literature (even though there are glaring and inexplicable omissions, as I have explained in earlier chapters), and they have made recommendations. But basically, I will always be skeptical toward official announcements, which I shall illustrate with an example from WHO.

I have studied in detail a WHO report from 2014 that seems to have been carried out in response to Aaby's findings of increased mortality of the trivalent diphtheria, tetanus, and pertussis (DTP) vaccine in Guinea-Bissau.[8] It assessed the effect of three vaccines on total mortality in infants and children: BCG, DTP, and measles.

I updated WHO's literature searches and found two highly relevant studies where Aaby and colleagues had improved on their previous research in response to the criticisms raised in the WHO report.[9] They found that the DTP vaccine doubled mortality, hazard ratio 2.14 (1.42 to 3.23), compared with DTP-unvaccinated children,[10] confirming their previous findings. In one of their studies, which represents the best available evidence, they explained that the criticisms raised in the WHO report were either not relevant, or they had taken it into account. They found that all the documented biases in their observational study favored the vaccinated group, i.e., they had likely underestimated the harmful effect of the DTP vaccine on mortality.

They also found that all studies of DTP that had analyzed existing data sets collected for other purposes suffered from substantial biases that led to underestimation of the harms of the vaccine. One such bias is frailty bias, where children with a poor prognosis generally tend to be vaccinated later or not at all. Another is survival bias. These studies have updated follow-up time for DTP-vaccinated children who survived, whereas children who died without their vaccination status being documented were classified as "unvaccinated." Such procedures introduce substantial bias and give a misleadingly high mortality rate in the unvaccinated group that makes it difficult to find a possible increase in mortality with DTP.

I found major problems with the WHO report. Although it reported that most studies showed a deleterious effect of DTP, the authors concluded that the results were inconsistent because two studies showed a beneficial effect. However, some heterogeneity will always occur in observational studies, and these two studies did not find a *significantly* beneficial effect on mortality. Furthermore, it was obvious that they were so seriously biased that they should not have been taken into account.

The authors did not provide summary estimates because WHO's working group had requested that meta-analyses not be done. This is an unacceptable interference with research by a body that includes people with numerous financial conflicts of interest in relation to vaccines. Furthermore, the reasons offered for not performing meta-analyses were invalid. It is difficult to understand why this highly unusual demand (which I have never seen elsewhere) was introduced unless one assumes that WHO did not want to run a risk of receiving a systematic review that suggested that the DTP vaccine increases total mortality.

WHO's experts who advised against using meta-analysis wrote, after having seen the WHO report, that the data suggested that both the BCG vaccine and the measles vaccine reduce all-cause mortality. I checked this claim by doing meta-analyses of the randomized trials that were included in the report, and I did not find significant reductions in mortality. Therefore, the experts could not conclude that these live attenuated vaccines reduce total mortality without also including the nonrandomized studies in their deliberations. In contrast, for the DTP vaccine they dismissed the nonrandomized studies. This is inconsistent and scientifically unacceptable, particularly considering that the results for the cohort studies for the BCG and the measles vaccines varied as much as those for the DTP vaccine.

I found many other serious problems with the WHO report. This is very surprising because two of the three authors of the WHO report are senior researchers in the Cochrane Collaboration. These two are the current editor-in-chief, Karla Soares-Weiser, and statistician Julian Higgins, who is editor of the 636-page *Cochrane Handbook*, which describes how to do reliable systematic reviews. These researchers even used vote counting in the WHO report (how many studies are for and how many against?), which is a method recommended against in the *Cochrane Handbook*.

A major problem with WHO is that the people who approved a vaccination program are also those who will consider whether there is reason to change their own recommendation. People are not likely to change their earlier decision, no matter how strong the evidence is that it was wrong.[11] Not a single randomized trial has been carried out, but the DTP vaccine is nonetheless on the market and is widely used.

Aaby and colleagues have pointed out that WHO even uses the DTP vaccine as a marker for good coverage of vaccination in general.[12] WHO has operated with reaching a "milestone of 90% national coverage" with three doses of the vaccine in all countries by 2015.[13] This should not happen. Program performance indicators should be those that are known to be positively associated with increased child survival.[14]

In addition to all this, we now have the odd situation that the burden of proof has been reversed. WHO recommends the use of the DTP vaccine and seems to require very convincing evidence that it increases mortality before any action will possibly be taken.

This is problematic. I consider Aaby's findings much more convincing than those in the WHO report, and we base our decisions on the best available evidence. This evidence tells us that the DTP vaccine likely increases total mortality in low-income countries. I therefore believe no one should be offered this vaccine without full informed consent that includes information that the vaccine is likely to increase total mortality. Furthermore, we need to do trials, e.g., where one of the groups receives a live vaccine shortly afterward.

Mumps

The mumps vaccine is usually given as part of the triple vaccine MMR. A systematic review of this vaccine did not find any randomized trials of the effect of the mumps component given separately, but cohort studies showed convincing effects.[15]

The effectiveness of at least one dose of MMR in preventing clinical mumps (as well as secondary mumps) in children was estimated to be around 75%.

The vaccine is so effective that very few people know what it is like to get mumps. I do because there was no vaccine when I was a child. The pain from my enlarged salivary glands was so intense that I cried a lot. I could not eat or smile without experiencing unendurable pain. I have also suffered tremendously from whooping cough, where I sounded like a sea lion. You never forget how horrible these diseases are once you have had them, and I wish the vaccine deniers knew about this.

There are also rare harms, of course, one of which is viral (aseptic) meningitis. The risk varies by a factor of 100 in different studies and surveys, ranging from 1 in 11,000 to 1 in a million.[16] However, even those that reported the largest risk, which was back in 1993 when the Urabe strain was still used (which I will discuss later), noted that the risk of getting meningitis from mumps was about fourfold higher for unvaccinated than for vaccinated people.[17] In addition, the vaccine risk might have been overestimated because it could be a chance laboratory finding in children investigated for other clinical conditions, particularly febrile convulsions.

It is reassuring that WHO reported in 2007 that no cases of virologically proven meningitis had been reported following the use of the Jeryl–Lynn strain (now very commonly used) or the RIT 4385 strain; that all reported cases of vaccine-derived mumps meningitis with other strains had recovered; and that some of these were laboratory diagnosed cases and had little, if any, clinical relevance.[18]

The Urabe strain has particularly often been identified in cases of viral meningitis, and this strain is therefore avoided. Already in 1990, the Trivarix measles, mumps, and rubella vaccine containing this strain was no longer licensed for sale in Canada.[19]

In conclusion, it is a terribly good idea to get vaccinated against mumps, which can lead to many harms including male infertility. But as usual, vaccine-denying websites are full of nonsense. One such site, with the seducing and misleading name "Child Health Safety," has a banner on its opening page with the text: "Vaccines did not save us—2 centuries of official statistics." It notes about itself that "This site aims to provide reliable information on child health safety for parents who want to know about whether they should vaccinate and other health related information."[20] This is false advertising, and the homepage even refers to the US Alliance for Human Research Protection, whose total lack of sense for truth-telling I described in Chapter 2.

In Child Health Safety's article about the mumps vaccine, Andrew Wakefield is mentioned 32 times, but I found nothing about his fraud.[21] The organization is secretive. I could not find any information on the website about the organization or its funders. I don't even know which country its leaders are based in or who they are. Funny that vaccine deniers so often accuse others of lack of transparency! When I googled *child health safety wordpress who are they*, the top hit was to a blogger who has analyzed some of the nonsense and misinformation propagated on the site.

Rubella

The systematic review did not identify any studies assessing the effectiveness of MMR in preventing rubella.[22]

Rubella is a mild viral infection, and the vaccine is primarily recommended to protect pregnant women in the first trimester because the infection can lead to fetal death, premature delivery, and serious birth defects.

The vaccine is highly effective. I could not find any information about its harms because it is always used as a component in the MMR vaccine. In its information about measles, the CDC noted that harms of the MMR vaccine include arthralgias and other joint symptoms, which are reported in up to 25% of susceptible adult women and are associated with the rubella component.[23] Other adverse events are subsequent mild illness, fever, a transient rash, and allergic reactions.

Polio

Vaccination against polio is one of the greatest triumphs of healthcare research. It is therefore not necessary to check any information about benefits and harms; we need the vaccine.

According to WHO,[24] poliomyelitis mainly affects children under 5 years of age, and 1 in 200 infections leads to irreversible paralysis. Among those paralyzed, 5% to 10% die when their breathing muscles become immobilized. Cases have decreased by over 99% since 1988, from an estimated 350,000 cases to 33 reported cases in 2018.

This is a highly harmful virus, and, as long as a single child remains infected, children in all countries are at risk of contracting polio if they are not vaccinated.

The vaccine exists both as a nonlive injected vaccine and as an oral attenuated vaccine (which many people have received on a piece of sugar). The attenuated vaccine causes a few outbreaks every year, e.g., in June 2017 it was reported that there had been 21 cases of vaccine-derived polio so far that year.[25] These cases are caused by remnants of the oral polio vaccine that have spread in the environment, mutated, and regained their ability to paralyze unvaccinated children. However, the live polio vaccine has saved a huge number of lives, and, like the measles vaccine, it seems to have strong, beneficial nonspecific effects.[26]

The outbreaks tend to happen in conflict zones where healthcare systems have collapsed, leaving many children unvaccinated, and they are also related to costs. The injectable vaccine—which is not live and therefore cannot mutate—is the one used in most developed countries, and it costs 30 times more than the oral polio vaccine used throughout most of the developing world.

Rotavirus

The rotavirus vaccine is not on the childhood vaccination program in my country even though we had a strong lobby group promoting it heavily. If you google *rotavirus program*, there are several interesting entries including a WHO report from 2013 that recommends that rotavirus vaccines be included in all national immunization programs and considered a priority, particularly in countries with high rotavirus gastroenteritis associated fatality rates, such as in South and Southeast Asia and sub-Saharan Africa.[27]

It is absolutely essential to ensure that the child is sufficiently hydrated, as dehydration is the cause of death. In Denmark, deaths due to rotavirus infection do not occur, which is the main reason why the vaccine is not part of our program. In the United States, there were around 3 million annual cases before the vaccine was introduced and 20–60 deaths.[28] These numbers cannot be compared to those in Europe because infant mortality is greater in the United States' privatized system, where many people cannot afford the healthcare they need.

It is clear that WHO went too far when it recommended this vaccination in all countries. And then there are the harms. The RotaShield vaccine was quickly withdrawn from the market when it was discovered that it often caused intussusception (which is a potentially lethal harm where the large intestine telescopes into itself).[29] A US research team estimated that the vaccine causes 1–2 additional cases of intussusception for every 10,000 infants vaccinated.[30] WHO has estimated that it is only 1–2 per 100,000 with the currently used vaccines.[31]

About half a million people die each year from rotavirus infections.[32] But does that justify a blanket recommendation to use the vaccine in all countries? What about establishing good sanitation, clean water, and ensuring the children are well hydrated, just like we do in cholera epidemics where these are the most important interventions? The vaccine is so expensive, at least in Denmark, that vaccinating 12 people corresponds to the gross domestic product per capita in Bangladesh. Who is going to pay for all this? Rich countries via donations, channeled from local governments to the vaccine manufacturers, GlaxoSmithKline and Merck,[33] which are already obscenely rich, have a business model that includes organized crime,[34] and over which we have no price control? That makes no sense to me.

Pneumococcal Infections

The most common infections caused by Streptococcus pneumoniae are otitis media (middle ear infection), sinusitis, and bronchitis; the most severe infections are pneumonia, meningitis, and sepsis. About 1.6 million people die of pneumococcal disease every year; around half of these are children aged less than five years, most of whom live in developing countries.[35]

The vaccines contain capsular polysaccharide antigens providing serotype-specific protection against the most serious infections; one of the currently marketed vaccines covers 23 serotypes, another 13, and a third 7.

A systematic review from 2009 included six randomized trials conducted in Africa, the Philippines, Finland, and the United States in infants up to two years of age, of which 57,015 received the vaccine, while 56,029 received placebo or another vaccine.[36] Vaccine efficacy for serotypes targeted by the vaccine was 80% (58% to 90%); for all serotypes 58% (29% to 75%); for X-ray confirmed pneumonia 27% (15% to 36%); and for all clinical pneumonias 6% (2% to 9%).

There was a nonsignificant reduction in all-cause mortality of 11% (-1% to 21%). This result was driven by a trial in The Gambia that carried 86% of the weight in the meta-analysis. It had a placebo control, which is reassuring given that the vaccine is nonlive and therefore expected to increase total mortality.

The other end of the age spectrum is also at increased risk for serious pneumococcal infections. A systematic review from 2013 that included 18 trials (64,852 adults) found that the vaccine reduced substantially the occurrence of invasive pneumococcal disease, odds ratio 0.26 (0.14 to 0.45), and all-cause pneumonia in low-income countries, odds ratio 0.54 (0.43 to 0.67), but not in high-income countries in either the general population, odds ratio 0.71 (0.45 to 1.12), or in adults with chronic illness, odds ratio 0.93 (0.73 to 1.19).[37] There was no statistically significant reduction in all-cause mortality, odds ratio 0.90 (0.74 to 1.09), and vaccine efficacy appeared to be poorer in adults with chronic illness.

It is not easy to make recommendations based on this, so let's see what the authorities made out of it. When I googled *pneumococcal vaccine recommendations*, the top link was to the CDC, which, unsurprisingly, recommended vaccination of the elderly: "CDC recommends 2 pneumococcal vaccines for all adults 65 years or older. You should receive a dose of PCV13 first, followed by a dose of PPSV23, at least 1 year later."[38] CDC also recommends the vaccine to all other adults if they have certain health conditions or smoke cigarettes. "Talk to your doctor to make sure you are up to date on these and other recommended vaccines." Okay, I have talked to my doctor, who is myself, and he says that I should *not* take the vaccine although I am over 65. We do not find the evidence compelling.

Even the CDC seems to have doubts. Farther down the first Google page, I found a note referring to a meeting from June 26, 2019:[39]

> In a narrow 8-6 vote today, a federal vaccine advisory panel shot down its 2014 recommendation that all adults 65 and older get a pneumococcal vaccine called Prevnar 13. Instead, the panel said seniors should get the vaccine based on conversations with their clinicians . . . to the dismay of the vaccine makers. Pfizer sells Prevnar 13, and the drug company's stock shot down 2% once investors learned of the vote. . . . Several members of the Advisory Committee on Immunization Practices, part of the Centers for Disease Control and Prevention, said this vote was one of the most difficult they've encountered.

The CDC only took a half-step back.[40] It was only the first of the recommended two doses that was now no longer recommended. The reason was that, since PCV13 was added to the childhood program in 2010, invasive disease in children has dropped by almost 80%. Through hugs and kisses and close association, children contributed their pneumococci to their elders, who now no longer got sick from those 13 strains. In addition, it turned out that the 2014 recommendation to vaccinate seniors had had no additional effect on disease rates.

I wonder why the CDC did not take a full step and also stopped recommending the 23-valent vaccine to seniors, when the full vaccination seems to have had no effect.

What this example demonstrates so nicely is that vaccine policies are based on assumptions that may quickly change and require new policies. In this way, vaccine policies are very different from all other policies in healthcare where the conditions are much more stable. The only exception is policies on the use of antibiotics, which may also need frequent updating, e.g., because of development of antibiotic resistance.

The Australian Department of Health has issued guidelines about who should be vaccinated according to age and whether they have any of a huge list of conditions that increase the risk of getting a pneumococcal infection or its severity.[41] These guidelines are overly bureaucratic, extremely complicated, and surely, no one will be able to remember all this. They look like a malicious joke and cannot possibly be evidence-based. They are worth reading because they are so utterly hopeless.

It is not easy to find anything about the harms of the vaccines, neither in the systematic reviews that did not look for them, nor on official websites that do not describe them. I googled *pneumococcal vaccine package insert*, and the first entry was to Pneumovax 23, Merck's 23-valent vaccine.[42] I would not exactly describe the harms as trivial. Already the first page has this information:

WARNINGS AND PRECAUTIONS: Use caution and appropriate care for individuals with severely compromised cardiovascular and/or pulmonary function in whom a systemic reaction would pose a significant risk.

ADVERSE REACTIONS: The most common adverse reactions, reported in >10% of subjects vaccinated with PNEUMOVAX 23 in clinical trials, were: injection-site pain/soreness/tenderness (60.0%), injection-site swelling/induration (20.3%), headache (17.6%), injection-site erythema (16.4%), asthenia and fatigue (13.2%), and myalgia (11.9%).

USE IN SPECIFIC POPULATIONS: Pregnancy: No human or animal data are available. Use only if clearly needed. Pediatrics: PNEUMOVAX 23 is not approved for use in children younger than 2 years of age because children in this age group do not develop an effective immune response to capsular types contained in the polysaccharide vaccine. Geriatrics: For subjects aged 65 years or older in a clinical study, systemic adverse reactions, determined by the investigator to be vaccine-related, were higher following revaccination (33.1%) than following initial vaccination (21.7%). Routine revaccination of immunocompetent persons previously vaccinated with a 23-valent vaccine, is not recommended.

DRUG INTERACTIONS: In a randomized clinical study, a reduced immune response to ZOSTAVAX° as measured by gpELISA was observed in individuals who received concurrent administration of PNEUMOVAX 23 and ZOSTAVAX compared with individuals who received these vaccines 4 weeks apart. Consider administration of the two vaccines separated by at least 4 weeks.

* * *

This is terribly interesting. I needed to write a whole book about vaccines before I found evidence that vaccines can interact negatively (see also Chapter 4). Zostavax is a live attenuated vaccine used to prevent shingles.

Farther down in the package insert, the harms are detailed, and we can see, for example, that "The proportion of subjects reporting injection site discomfort that interfered with or prevented usual activity or injection site induration ≥4 inches was higher following revaccination (30.6%) than following initial vaccination (10.4%). Injection site reactions typically resolved by 5 days following vaccination."[43] Typically resolved within 5 days? What happened to those who were less fortunate, and how long did it take for them to recover from the vaccine?

You can read more about adverse effects, which will not increase your appetite for getting this vaccine. A colossal amount of people will be harmed for everyone who will benefit (if anyone will, as mentioned). Not a vaccine that will ever come on my menu. Why does the CDC and WHO not give us such essential information?

You may look up information in the same way as I did if you wish to find out what the harms are of other vaccines. The 13-valent vaccine (Prevnar 13) is currently used in Denmark for small children, and the package insert is not particularly persuasive if you consider getting your child vaccinated:

> In infants and toddlers vaccinated at 2, 4, 6, and 12-15 months of age in US clinical trials, the most commonly reported solicited adverse reactions (>5%) were irritability (>70%), injection site tenderness (>50%), decreased appetite (>40%), decreased sleep (>40%), increased sleep (>40%), fever (>20%), injection site redness (>20%), and injection site swelling (>20%).[44]

In Denmark, infants have been vaccinated since 2007. Invasive infection with nonvaccine serotypes have increased, but totally, the incidence of invasive infection in the whole population has decreased from 20 to 15 per 100,000[45]

I have been unable to find data on number of deaths, but when vaccination of infants was introduced, it was estimated that it would save one life per year in Danish children below 5 years of age.[46]

Thus, although fewer deaths among the elderly are expected due to vaccination of the infants, the effect of vaccinating the whole population (about 60,000 children are born each year in Denmark) is very small. It can be discussed whether this is worthwhile, also compared to what else we might do. We all know how it feels to get a virus infection. A serious bacterial infection feels different, and the person may not realize how dangerous the situation is, or that it is caused by a bacterium. Therefore, if people go to their doctors when they feel diffusely unwell, not like themselves, and appropriate tests are carried out, e.g., a blood culture and a throat swab, I think many deaths could be avoided by earlier intervention with antibiotics.

Meningitis Caused by Meningococci

It is of utmost importance to see a doctor as quickly as possible if you suspect that you could have bacterial meningitis caused by meningococci, or sepsis with meningococci. The difference between life and death can be a matter of minutes. Most deaths could be avoided if this precaution were adhered to, and if the patient or the parents refuse being sent back home with a reassuring message that all will be fine when they feel that all is *not* fine.[47]

Even though this is a book about vaccines, this is worth mentioning: meningitis is often misinterpreted as being something else. What you should particularly look out for is leg pains, cold hands and feet, and abnormal skin color. These are signs of sepsis. The classic symptoms and signs such as hemorrhagic rash (small spots with bleeding in the skin), meningism (neck stiffness, intolerance to bright light and headaches), and impaired consciousness develop about eight hours later, on average, which may be too late for antibiotics to work.

In some areas in the world, e.g., in sub-Saharan Africa in the Sahel belt, epidemics of meningitis occur, and it can be very wise to vaccinate the populations. It is more uncertain in the Western world, as illustrated by the conflicting advice given in different countries of similar standing. Very few people die from infections with meningococci in these countries, which is the main reason why policies differ.

Hepatitis

No globally valid recommendations can be made because the risk of getting hepatitis varies hugely between countries. WHO has estimated that about 780,000 people die each year due to the consequences of hepatitis B, such as liver cirrhosis and liver cancer. It recommends that all infants receive their first dose of vaccine as soon as possible after birth.[48]

In Denmark, where the disease is rare, we only recommend vaccination of certain risk groups, e.g., drug abusers and sex partners of infected people, or if people are planning a longer stay in areas where the disease is common.

For hepatitis A, vaccination is recommended when traveling to areas where the disease is common, which may include southern Europe. It can be pretty serious to acquire the infection, which can cause extreme fatigue for months. Unlike hepatitis B and C, hepatitis A infection does not cause chronic liver disease and is very rarely fatal (due to acute liver failure). There are only about 35 cases in Denmark each year. The disease is usually transmitted via drinking water and food, and in 2015, there was an outbreak due to imported strawberries from North Africa.

Varicella

Chicken pox is a highly contagious disease that is much milder than measles, another highly contagious disease. Before vaccinations became available, the case fatality rates for varicella were only about one-hundredth of that for measles.[49] Varicella tends to be more severe in adults because they usually get the infection from their own child.

Following infection, the virus remains latent in neural ganglia. Upon subsequent reactivation, the varicella zoster virus may cause shingles (herpes zoster), which mainly affects immunocompromised and elderly people. The unilateral vesicular rash, characteristically restricted to a single dermatome (skin area innervated by one nerve), is usually accompanied by radicular pain and discomfort that may last for weeks, months, or even years.

The vaccines are live attenuated ones. WHO does not recommend universal vaccination but suggests routine childhood immunization in countries where the disease has an important public health impact.[50]

Other Vaccines

Smallpox

A book about vaccines should mention one of the biggest successes in medical history, the eradication of smallpox, which was officially declared by WHO in 1980.[1] Only ten years earlier, the last patient died from smallpox in Denmark.[2] It was a young Norwegian who studied in Copenhagen. He had been to Afghanistan, and a few days after his return, he was admitted to the hospital with severe symptoms of smallpox. The whole country was immediately put on the alert because smallpox is highly contagious. If an epidemic broke out, airports would be closed and there would be huge losses for the national economy.

An intensive search started for possible secondary cases, which was a formidable task, as the patient had been extremely social. It was estimated that the patient had been in contact with 689 people since his return, which included foreigners about to leave Denmark and people who were not vaccinated for religious reasons. However, thanks to well-coordinated searches that involved Interpol, all the possibly infected people were located within a week.

They were isolated in tent camps in the hospital area for two weeks. Miraculously, none of them developed smallpox, which no one could explain. But the patient died.

Seventeen years later, when I took the history of a newly admitted Danish woman at the same department of infectious diseases, I was told she had had smallpox as a child. Somewhat skeptical, I asked: "I suppose you mean varicella?" But no, she was isolated at the age of five and remembered that her parents were only allowed to see her through a glass window in the door.

Smallpox is a horrible disease although it also exists in less virulent forms. The death rate is about 30%; many of those who survive have extensive scarring of their skin; and in epidemics, one-third may be left blind.[3] Smallpox is estimated to have killed around 500 million people in the last 100 years of its existence, and as recently as 1967, 15 million cases occurred a year. Parents did not know whether their children would survive childhood before they had had smallpox.

In wars, smallpox has often played a prominent role. The Spanish sailors brought the disease with them when they conquered Central America in the sixteenth century, and it killed most of the native people. During the French-German war in 1870–71, more than 23,000 French soldiers died of smallpox compared to only 300 German soldiers, because the Germans had been more thorough with vaccinating their soldiers.

Smallpox gives us a historical perspective on vaccines. The smallpox vaccine was the first vaccine ever used and has also been one of the most successful ones. Prevention of smallpox had been carried out for centuries in Asia and the Middle East, where children were inoculated with a mild form of the disease to make them immune, before the method came to Europe in the 1700s and became standard practice in England.[4] Inoculation involved introducing material from smallpox pustules into the skin, which generally produced a less severe infection than naturally acquired smallpox yet still induced immunity to it.

However, it involved serious risks—both to the recipient and others—because those inoculated could pass on the disease after becoming carriers.[5]

In the 1700s, it was common knowledge among the rural population that milkmaids and other people who had developed cowpox were spared during smallpox epidemics. This cross immunity also meant that milkmaids were prettier than other girls because their faces were not scarred. In 1798, Edward Jenner, a physician and scientist who had practiced vaccination for some years, applied for permission to present his results to the Royal Society in London. His request was refused because "he ought not to risk his reputation by presenting to the learned body anything which appeared so much at variance with established knowledge and withal so incredible."[6] However, as is often the case in the history of medicine, the established knowledge was wrong, the "non-learned body"—ordinary people in the countryside—was correct, and this new preventive treatment soon received widespread acceptance.

Based on historical data, smallpox vaccination causes about one death per million persons.[7] Deaths have also occurred among nonvaccinated persons who had accidental contact with vaccination sites of vaccine recipients, and vaccination of pregnant women can cause stillbirth or infant death.

The Latin word for cow is *vacca*, and Jenner called cowpox *Variolae vaccinae*, which is how the term vaccination originated. The term smallpox was first used in Britain in the fifteenth century to distinguish the disease from syphilis, which was then known as the great pox.

Yellow fever

Yellow fever is a viral disease of typically short duration, but in about 15% of people, the liver is affected, which causes the skin to turn yellow and increases the risk of bleeding and kidney problems.[8]

As for malaria, mosquito control plays a major role in disease prevention because yellow fever is transmitted by mosquitoes. It infects only humans and other primates, and outbreaks have occurred in relation to deforestation when the monkeys are brought down from the canopy.

The disease originated in Africa and spread to South America with the slave trade. It is common in tropical areas in South America and Africa, but not in Asia. In 2013, yellow fever resulted in about 127,000 severe infections and 45,000 deaths, with nearly 90% of these occurring in Africa.

Should you get vaccinated if you live in an area where the disease occurs or visits such an area?

Let's look at the harms of the vaccine first. Serious harms of the attenuated live vaccine are very rare.[9] One person per 200,000 doses develops a disease similar to yellow fever within a week of vaccination, with fever, muscle pain, nausea, vomiting, and diarrhea, which can progress to multisystem organ failure and death. More than 60 cases worldwide have been reported to the CDC of which two-thirds of the victims died.

Another very rare reaction (less than one case per 100,000 doses) is neurologic disease, which includes meningoencephalitis (inflammation of the brain and its membranes), Guillain-Barré syndrome, acute disseminated encephalomyelitis (inflammation of the brain and spinal cord), and paralysis of the motor units of the cranial nerves. In rare cases, these reactions are fatal.

These vaccine-induced diseases are more common in persons aged 60 years or older. These ages are therefore considered a precaution to receiving the vaccine in the United States, where the vaccine is recommended only for travelers who plan to visit areas where the disease is present and for laboratory personnel who work with yellow fever virus.[10]

In areas where yellow fever is common, early diagnosis of cases and immunization of large parts of the population are important to prevent outbreaks.[11]

In some cases, you have no choice other than being vaccinated because some countries require vaccinations for travelers. In other cases, you might wish to do an assessment similar to the one I described in the chapter about Japanese encephalitis. Or, you could simply trust the authorities because countries that are less prone to recommend vaccines than the United States also recommend the vaccine to travelers to infected areas.

Dengue

Dengue is a mosquito-borne tropical disease. The dengue virus causes mild, flu-like symptoms in most people, but rarely, patients develop severe disease, with potentially fatal bleeding and organ damage. As something extremely unusual, the risk of severe disease is higher in people who have been infected a second time.

The vaccine Dengvaxia contains attenuated yellow fever viruses that have been manipulated so that they contain proteins from dengue virus. It protects against four serotypes. According to EMA, it is only for use in people from 9 to 45 years of age who have been infected with dengue virus (confirmed by a laboratory test) before and who live in areas where the disease occurs regularly throughout the year.[12]

Three trials have been carried out in Asia and Latin America involving over 35,000 children. The trials included both children who had and had not been infected with dengue virus before. Overall, among children aged 9 to 16 years who had had previous dengue infection, there were around 79% fewer cases of dengue disease compared with placebo.[13] However, in children who had not had previous dengue infection, the risk of severe disease if they later became infected was higher in those vaccinated than in those given placebo (two additional cases per 1,000 people vaccinated over 5 years). The vaccine also had only 39% effect in these people.[14] Additional studies showed that the vaccine is also effective in people aged 16 to 45 years.

The most common adverse effects of Dengvaxia (which occur in more than 10% of the vaccinees) are headache, injection site pain, malaise (feeling unwell), muscle pain, weakness, and fever. Allergic reactions, which may be severe, are very rare.

Recent events in the Philippines are interesting, both for vaccines in general and for the controversial issue of mandatory vaccinations. Dengvaxia was first licensed in Mexico, in December 2015, for use in people 9–45 years of age.[15] At the same time, former President Benigno Aquino III met with executives of Sanofi Pasteur in a courtesy call in Paris, making the Philippines the first Asian country to approve Dengvaxia, and a school-based immunization program was quickly launched.[16]

Two years later, the Philippine Department of Health suspended the vaccination program following a press release by Sanofi Pasteur that noted that the vaccine might worsen the disease if the recipient had not had it earlier. A little later, the Philippine Food and Drug Administration ordered Sanofi to stop selling Dengvaxia. A medical director of Sanofi said that the dengue vaccination would not cause severe dengue, but another Sanofi representative needed to apologize during a hearing in the House of Representatives.

There were also countermovements. A group of doctors, including a former health minister, urged the Public Attorney's Office to stop conducting autopsies, and Aquino said the controversy had been "politicized."

A Philippine newspaper reported that the chair of the Senate Committee on Health and Demography wanted to investigate if there had been an "irregularity" in the procurement of the vaccine. In April 2018, a senator released his draft report of the issues stating that Aquino was guilty of "malfeasance, misfeasance and nonfeasance." The Public Attorney's Office filed criminal charges about reckless imprudence resulting in homicide against former Health Minister Janette Garin and other officials. Some of the parents of the dead children had no prior knowledge of their children being vaccinated, and some families also filed charges.

A year later, the Department of Justice recommended the charges be filed in court and stated that the government registered and bought Dengvaxia for its immunization program with undue haste.[17] Six Sanofi officials, 14 current and former Philippine health officials, and previous Minister Janette Garin would be charged.

Sanofi said, "We strongly disagree with the findings made against Sanofi and some of its employees and we will vigorously defend them." This is the standard script when a drug company has brought itself into trouble. Only one month earlier, the Philippines had revoked the product's license after concluding Sanofi had failed to meet directives issued by regulators.

There were 35 deaths under investigation, but the head of the panel of medical experts noted that medical records of 119 victims would be examined.

The public prosecutors said that 20 officials had shown neglect in having "totally disregarded the identified risks and adverse effects of the vaccine." They also said Sanofi had failed to closely monitor the recipients of Dengvaxia, nor did it extend medical assistance to victims or their families, even after reports of serious adverse reactions surfaced.

Rabies

People are very different in terms of the risks they are willing to take, which is why we decide differently given the same evidence. For instance, although rabies is extremely rare, I would get vaccinated for rabies if bitten by a dog, or a wild animal in tropical countries or in North America. You should be particularly cautious with bats, e.g., vampire bats, which live in Central and South America, can bite you while you are asleep without waking you up. It takes several weeks for rabies to kill you, and postexposure vaccination is highly effective.

Rabies is one of the extremely rare occurrences in medicine where only one patient is enough to convince us that an intervention is effective. When Louis Pasteur in 1885 gave a rabies vaccination to a boy who had been bitten multiple times by a rabid dog, and he survived, the scientist was convinced that the vaccine had worked because rabies is considered fatal.

10

Conclusions about Vaccines

WHO has listed reluctance or refusal to vaccinate as one of the top ten global health threats that run the risk of reversing progress made in tackling vaccine-preventable diseases.[1] WHO has estimated that vaccination is one of the most cost-effective ways of avoiding disease. Vaccinations prevent 2–3 million deaths a year, and a further 1.5 million deaths could be avoided if global coverage of vaccinations improved.

Vaccines differ markedly in their benefits and harms, and for some, it can be questioned whether they are worthwhile using. We therefore need to study carefully each vaccine separately if we want to arrive at a rational decision whether we should get vaccinated or should have our children vaccinated.

Some people, around 1–2% in high-income countries,[2] are opposed to all vaccines, as if there were no differences between them. If anyone wants to speak about vaccines in a general way, without differentiating between them, the scientific facts are very convincing: it is vastly better to get all the recommended vaccines than to refuse all of them. It is far more likely that we will be seriously or fatally injured by diseases that could have been prevented by vaccines than by the vaccines themselves.

However, we can do much better than to simply accept everything that is recommended. Recommendations vary considerably from country to country of similar standing (Chapter 8), which means that some vaccines are not that important. Furthermore, people with an influence on guidelines often have financial conflicts of interest in relation to the vaccine industry. Even when there are no such issues, the authorities sometimes spread information that is seriously misleading. After having read what the

CDC writes about flu shots, I don't trust anything this agency writes about the necessity of being vaccinated.

It has been abundantly documented that we cannot trust the drug agencies, either.[3] In their work, they rely far too much on what drug companies tell them even though they know very well that fraud, bias, and underreporting of serious drug harms in industry-sponsored drug trials are common.[4] It cannot be repeated often enough that our prescription drugs are the third-leading cause of death,[5] which demonstrates that drug agencies are dysfunctional; they do not protect us against lethal harms of drugs. Nonetheless, package inserts approved by drug agencies are useful sources of information when we try to find out what the harms of vaccines are.

I have mixed feelings about WHO. There are far too many issues with financial conflicts of interest, and there have been too many unfortunate announcements and recommendations, e.g., the declaration of a flu pandemic in 2009 that proved to be milder than other influenza epidemics and the associated stockpiling of Tamiflu, and the new criteria for vaccine harms that make it virtually impossible to ever conclude that a vaccine causes a suspected harm (Chapter 6).

I have argued why I am against mandatory vaccinations (Chapter 3). But I must admit that the threat to other people, not least people's own children who cannot make decisions about vaccines for themselves, might become so large that I would favor mandatory vaccinations of some kind. Hopefully without using force, which I find repugnant.

There is far too much we don't know about vaccines, and it is too easy to get them approved based on substandard trials conducted by the manufacturers with no placebo controls, where many harms are never recorded or are suppressed, and where the authority on top of this erroneously claims that the vaccine adjuvants are safe (Chapter 6).

We know virtually nothing about what happens when we use many vaccines and about their long-term effects on the immune system, and it is shocking that I needed to write a whole book about vaccines before I found evidence that vaccines can interact negatively (Chapters 4 and 8). If we study vaccines more closely, there will be other unexpected revelations, and I have mentioned some of those. For example, flu shots likely increase the risk of getting influenza with other strains, compared to people who are not vaccinated;[6] the dengue vaccine should be avoided if people have not already had dengue in the past because the risk of severe disease is too great (Chapter 9); nonlive vaccines may increase total mortality, whereas live attenuated vaccines may decrease total mortality; and the sequence of the vaccines and the sex of the recipient also seem to matter (Chapter 1).

Billions of people are being vaccinated and billions are being earned on vaccines. There is no excuse for not demanding much more rigorous trials, including proper testing of the safety of the adjuvants. Large trials with long follow-up that allows registration of late-occurring harms should be carried out independently of the drug industry, financed by the public purse. They need not be expensive, as they could be simple and pragmatic, with a minimum of administrative costs. They will likely be cost-effective, as we will likely find out that some vaccines or their combinations should be avoided.

It is of vital importance to ensure that issues about vaccines be discussed openly, without harassment, and that no one avoid registering suspected harms in vaccine trials or clinical practice out of fear of repercussions, including public humiliation or worse, loss of job, which happened to me in large part because I criticized the prestigious but poorly done Cochrane review of the HPV vaccines (Chapter 6).[7]

My final remark is about political expediency. To make promises about new offerings in healthcare—whether they work or not is immaterial—can give you many votes and may ensure that your party be represented in the next government. Two weeks before the elections that made Margaret Thatcher prime minister in the United Kingdom, she promised to introduce mammography screening.

The rest follows from there. Everyone in a leading position in healthcare knows what is expected of them if they want to be popular with the politicians. You don't get popular by raising critical questions about vaccines.

About the Author

Professor Peter C. Gøtzsche graduated as a Master of Science in biology and chemistry in 1974 and as a physician 1984. He is a specialist in internal medicine and worked with clinical trials and regulatory affairs in the drug industry from 1975 to 1983, and at hospitals in Copenhagen from 1984 to 1995. With about 80 others, he cofounded the Cochrane Collaboration in 1993 (the founder is Sir Iain Chalmers) and established the Nordic Cochrane Centre the same year. He became professor of Clinical Research Design and Analysis in 2010 at the University of Copenhagen and has been a member of the Cochrane Governing Board twice. He now works freelance. He became visiting professor, Institute of Health & Society, Newcastle University in 2019 and founded the Institute for Scientific Freedom in the same year.

Gøtzsche has published more than 75 papers in "the big five" (*BMJ*, *Lancet*, *JAMA*, *Annals of Internal Medicine*, and *New England Journal of Medicine*), and his scientific works have been cited over 150,000 times. His most recent books are:

- *Mental health survival kit and withdrawal from psychiatric drugs* (2020).
- *Survival in an overmedicated world: look up the evidence yourself* (2019).
- *Death of a whistleblower and Cochrane's moral collapse* (2019).
- *Deadly psychiatry and organised denial* (2015).
- *Deadly medicines and organised crime: How big pharma has corrupted health care* (2013) (Winner, British Medical Association's Annual Book Award in the category Basis of Medicine in 2014).
- *Mammography screening: truth, lies and controversy* (2012) (Winner of the Prescrire Prize 2012).
- *Rational diagnosis and treatment: evidence-based clinical decision-making* (2007).

Four of these books have appeared in multiple languages; see deadlymedi-cines.dk.

Gøtzsche has given numerous interviews, one of which, about organized crime in the drug industry, has been seen over 400,000 times on YouTube: https://www.youtube.com/watch?v=dozpAshvtsA. He appeared on *The Daily Show* in New York on Sept. 16, 2014, where he played the role of Deep Throat, revealing secrets about big pharma. A documentary film about his reform work in psychiatry, *Diagnosing Psychiatry*, appeared in 2017.

He has an interest in statistics and research methodology. He has coauthored the following guidelines for good reporting of research: CONSORT for randomised trials (www.consort-statement.org), STROBE for observational studies (www.strobe-statement.org), PRISMA for system-atic reviews and meta-analyses (www.prisma-statement.org), and SPIRIT for trial protocols (www.spirit-statement.org).

Gøtzsche is Protector for the Hearing Voices Network in Denmark.

Websites: scientificfreedom.dk and deadlymedicines.dk

Twitter: @PGtzsche1

Notes

CHAPTER 1

[1] Mohdin A. Matt Hancock 'won't rule out' compulsory vaccinations. *The Guardian* 2019; May.

[2] Moyer MW. Anti-vaccine activists have taken vaccine science hostage. *New York Times* 2018; Aug. 4.

[3] Ibid.

[4] Skowronski DM, De Serres G, Crowcroft NS, et al. Association between the 2008–09 seasonal influenza vaccine and pandemic H1N1 illness during spring–summer 2009: four observational studies from Canada. *PLoS Med* 2010;7:e1000258.

[5] Moyer MW. Anti-vaccine activists have taken vaccine science hostage.

[6] Witczak K. Vaccine controversy: Why can't we just have a conversation instead of name calling? 2019; Apr. 26. https://www.linkedin.com/pulse/vaccine-controversy-why-cant -we-just-have-instead-name-kim-witczak/.

[7] Gøtzsche PC. *Deadly psychiatry and organised denial.* Copenhagen: People's Press; 2015.

[8] Ibid.

[9] Witczak K. Vaccine controversy: Why can't we just have a conversation instead of name calling?

[10] Gøtzsche PC. *Deadly psychiatry and organised denial.*

[11] Ibid; Gøtzsche PC. *Deadly medicines and organised crime: How big pharma has corrupted health care.* London: Radcliffe Publishing; 2013.

[12] Ibid.

[13] https://icandecide.org/government/FDA-Production-FOIA.pdf.

[14] Benn CS, Fisker AB, Aaby P (eds.). Bandim Health Project, 1978–2018. Forty years of contradicting conventional wisdom. Contact: bandim@ssi.dk. All publications are available at https://www.bandim.org/publications.aspx.

[15] Aaby P, Ravn H, Benn CS. The WHO review of the possible nonspecific effects of diphtheria-tetanus-pertussis vaccine. *Pediatr Infect Dis J* 2016;35:1247–57; Mogensen SW, Andersen A, Rodrigues A, et al. The introduction of diphtheria-tetanus-pertussis and oral polio vaccine among young infants in an urban African community: a natural experiment. *EBioMedicine* 2017;17:192–8.

[16] Gøtzsche PC. *Death of a whistleblower and Cochrane's moral collapse.* Copenhagen: People's Press; 2019.

[17] Sarlin J. Anti-vaccination conspiracy theories thrive on Amazon. CNN 2019; Feb. 27.

[18] Wong JC. How Facebook and YouTube help spread anti-vaxxer propaganda. *The Guardian* 2019; Feb. 1.

[19] Ibid.

[20] Ibid.

[21] Gøtzsche PC. *Survival in an overmedicated world: look up the evidence yourself.* Copenhagen: People's Press; 2019.

[22] Editorial Board. How to Inoculate Against Anti-Vaxxers. *New York Times* 2019; Jan. 19.

[23] Ibid.

[24] Moran M, Everhart K, Lucas M, et al. Why are anti-vaccine messages so persuasive? A content analysis of anti-vaccine websites to inform the development of vaccine promotion strategies. 2015; Nov. 3. https://apha.confex.com/apha/143am/webprogram /Paper329083.html.

[25] Gøtzsche PC. *Survival in an overmedicated world: look up the evidence yourself.*

[26] Pilkington E, Glenza J. Facebook under pressure to halt rise of anti-vaccination groups. *The Guardian* 2019; Feb. 12.

[27] Gøtzsche PC. *Survival in an overmedicated world: look up the evidence yourself.*

[28] Ibid.

[29] Pilkington E, Glenza J. Facebook under pressure to halt rise of anti-vaccination groups.

[30] Editorial Board. How to Inoculate Against Anti-Vaxxers.

[31] Ibid.

[32] Gøtzsche PC. *Deadly medicines and organised crime: How big pharma has corrupted health care.*

[33] Gøtzsche PC. *Deadly psychiatry and organised denial.*

[34] Miller ER, Moro PL, Cano M, et al. Deaths following vaccination: What does the evidence show? *Vaccine* 2015;33:3288–92.

[35] Ibid.

[36] Ibid.

[37] Ibid.

[38] Ibid.

[39] Gøtzsche PC. *Deadly medicines and organised crime: How big pharma has corrupted health care.*

[40] Ibid.

[41] National Academies of Sciences, Engineering, and Medicine. Adverse effects of vaccines: evidence and causality. 2011. http://www.nationalacademies.org/hmd/Reports/2011 /Adverse-Effects-of-Vaccines-Evidence-and-Causality.aspx.

[42] Miller ER, Moro PL, Cano M, et al. Deaths following vaccination: What does the evidence show?

[43] Ibid.

[44] Ibid.

[45] Doshi P. The unofficial vaccine educators: are CDC funded non-profits sufficiently independent? *BMJ* 2017;359:j5104.

[46] Ibid.

[47] Ibid.

[48] Ibid.

[49] Pedante I, Dal Monte PP. *Immunità di legge. I vaccini obbligatori tra scienza al governo e governo della scienza.* Bologna: Ariana Editrice; 2018.

[50] Ibid.

[51] Ibid.

[52] Paulson T. Doctors Without Borders criticizes Gates-backed global vaccine strategy. 2012; May 15. http://www.humanosphere.org/global-health/2012/05/doctors-without -borders-criticizes-gates-backed-global-vaccine-strategy/.

CHAPTER 2

[1] Aaby P. Malnourished or overinfected. An analysis of the determinants of acute measles mortality. *Dan Med Bull* 1989;36:93–113.

[2] Aaby P. Severe measles in Copenhagen, 1915–1925. Rev Infect Dis 1988;10:452–6.

[3] World Health Organization. Measles. 2018; Nov. 29. https://www.who.int/en/news -room/fact-sheets/detail/measles.

[4] Ibid.

[5] Prof. Peter Gøtzsche (@PGtzsche1), Tweet, February 17, 2019. https://twitter.com /pgtzsche1/status/1097057069428080640?lang=en.

[6] David Gorski (@gorskon), Tweet, February 15, 2019. https://twitter.com/gorskon /status/1096391877094502402.

[7] Dachel A. AofA Q&A: Dr. Toni Bark Illinois MD on pediatric health and vaccination status. 2014; Nov. 3. https://www.ageofautism.com/2014/11/aofa-qa-dr-toni-bark-illinois -md-on-pediatric-health-and-vaccination-status.html.

[8] Holland M. Who is Dr. Andrew Wakefield? Chapter 28. http://vaxxedthemovie.com /wp-content/uploads/2016/04/Who-is-Dr.-Andrew-Wakefield-by-Mary-Holland-JD .pdf.

[9] Deer B. How the case against the MMR vaccine was fixed. *BMJ* 2011;342:c5347; Deer B. The Lancet's two days to bury bad news. *BMJ* 2011;342:c7001; Deer B. How the vaccine crisis was meant to make money. *BMJ* 2011;342:c5258; Deer B. Who saw the "histological findings"? *BMJ* 2011;343:d7892; Deer B. Pathology reports solve "new bowel disease" riddle. *BMJ* 2011;343:d6823; Godlee F, Smith J, Marcovitch H. Wakefield's article linking MMR vaccine and autism was fraudulent. *BMJ* 2011;342:c7452; Godlee F. Institutional and editorial misconduct in the MMR scare. *BMJ* 2011;342:d378; Deer B. Andrew Wakefield concocts a conspiracy. Undated. http://briandeer.com/solved/tall -story.htm.

[10] Godlee F, Smith J, Marcovitch H. Wakefield's article linking MMR vaccine and autism was fraudulent.

[11] https://www.scientificfreedom.dk/. There is a link on the front page to presentations at the symposium March 9, 2019.

[12] Deer B. How the case against the MMR vaccine was fixed; Deer B. The Lancet's two days to bury bad news; Deer B. How the vaccine crisis was meant to make money; Deer B. Who saw the "histological findings"?; Deer B. Pathology reports solve "new bowel disease" riddle; Godlee F, Smith J, Marcovitch H. Wakefield's article linking MMR vaccine and autism was fraudulent; Godlee F. Institutional and editorial misconduct in the MMR scare; Deer B. Andrew Wakefield concocts a conspiracy.

[13] Wakefield AJ, Murch SH, Anthony A, et al. Ileal-lymphoid-nodular hyperplasia, non-specific colitis, and pervasive developmental disorder in children. *Lancet* 1998;351:637–41.

[14] Deer B. How the case against the MMR vaccine was fixed; Deer B. The Lancet's two days to bury bad news; Deer B. How the vaccine crisis was meant to make money; Deer

B. Who saw the "histological findings"?; Deer B. Pathology reports solve "new bowel disease" riddle; Godlee F, Smith J, Marcovitch H. Wakefield's article linking MMR vaccine and autism was fraudulent; Godlee F. Institutional and editorial misconduct in the MMR scare

15 "Andrew Wakefield: the fraud investigation," https://briandeer.com/mmr/lancet -summary.htm.

16 Deer B. How the vaccine crisis was meant to make money; "Andrew Wakefield: the fraud investigation."

17 Deer B. How the vaccine crisis was meant to make money.

18 "Andrew Wakefield: the fraud investigation."

19 Wakefield AJ, Murch SH, Anthony A, et al. Ileal-lymphoid-nodular hyperplasia, non-specific colitis, and pervasive developmental disorder in children.

20 "Andrew Wakefield: the fraud investigation."

21 Ibid.

22 Ibid.

23 Ibid.

24 Deer B. How the case against the MMR vaccine was fixed; "Andrew Wakefield: the fraud investigation."

25 Deer B. The Lancet's two days to bury bad news.

26 Ibid.

27 Ibid.

28 Ibid.

29 Murch SH, Anthony A, Casson DH, et al. Retraction of an interpretation. *Lancet* 2004;363:750.

30 Godlee F, Smith J, Marcovitch H. Wakefield's article linking MMR vaccine and autism was fraudulent; Godlee F. Institutional and editorial misconduct in the MMR scare.

31 Godlee F, Smith J, Marcovitch H. Wakefield's article linking MMR vaccine and autism was fraudulent.

32 Flaherty DK. The vaccine-autism connection: a public health crisis caused by unethical medical practices and fraudulent science. *Ann Pharmacother* 2011;45:1302–4.

33 Ibid.

34 Deer B. How the case against the MMR vaccine was fixed; Deer B. The Lancet's two days to bury bad news; Deer B. How the vaccine crisis was meant to make money; Deer B. Who saw the "histological findings"?; Deer B. Pathology reports solve "new bowel disease" riddle; Godlee F, Smith J, Marcovitch H. Wakefield's article linking MMR vaccine and autism was fraudulent; Godlee F. Institutional and editorial misconduct in the MMR scare

35 Brogan K. CDC: You're fired. Autism coverup exposed. Undated; the first comment is from 2014. https://kellybroganmd.com/cdc-youre-fired-autism-coverup-exposed/.

36 DeStefano F, Bhasin TK, Thompson WW, et al. Age at first measles-mumps-rubella vaccination in children with autism and school-matched control subjects: a population-based study in metropolitan Atlanta. *Pediatrics* 2004;113:259–66.

37 Hooker BS. Measles-mumps-rubella vaccination timing and autism among young African American boys: a reanalysis of CDC data. *Transl Neurodegener* 2014;3:16. RETRACTED.

38 DeStefano F, Bhasin TK, Thompson WW, et al. Age at first measles-mumps-rubella vaccination in children with autism and school-matched control subjects: a population-based study in metropolitan Atlanta.

39 Taubes G. Epidemiology faces its limits. *Science* 1995;269:164–9.

40 Madsen KM, Hviid A, Vestergaard M, et al. A population-based study of measles, mumps, and rubella vaccination and autism. *N Engl J Med* 2002;347:1477–82.

41 Hooker BS. Measles-mumps-rubella vaccination timing and autism among young African American boys: a reanalysis of CDC data.

42 DeStefano F, Bhasin TK, Thompson WW, et al. Age at first measles-mumps-rubella vaccination in children with autism and school-matched control subjects: a population-based study in metropolitan Atlanta.

43 Ibid.

44 Hooker BS. Measles-mumps-rubella vaccination timing and autism among young African American boys: a reanalysis of CDC data.

45 Orac. Vaxxed: From cover-up to catastrophe. 2016; July 18. https://respectfulinsolence .com/2016/07/18/in-which-andrew-wakefield-and-del-bigtrees-antivaccine -documentary-vaxxed-is-reviewed-with-insolence/.

46 Ibid.

47 Gøtzsche PC. *Survival in an overmedicated world: look up the evidence yourself.* Copenhagen: People's Press; 2019.

48 Orac. Vaxxed: From cover-up to catastrophe.

49 Boseley S. How disgraced anti-vaxxer Andrew Wakefield was embraced by Trump's America. *The Guardian* 2018; July 18.

50 "Press Awards 2011: The full list of winners," *Press Gazette*, April 5, 2011, https://www .pressgazette.co.uk/press-awards-2011-the-full-list-of-winners/.

51 Verstraeten T, Davis RL, DeStefano F. Increased risk of developmental neurologic impairment after high exposure to thimerosal-containing vaccine in first month of life. Abstract at EIS Conference; 1999.

52 Verstraeten T, Davis RL, DeStefano F, et al. Safety of thimerosal-containing vaccines: a two-phased study of computerized health maintenance organization databases. *Pediatrics* 2003;112:1039–48.

53 Madsen KM, Hviid A, Vestergaard M, et al. A population-based study of measles, mumps, and rubella vaccination and autism; Madsen KM, Lauritsen MB, Pedersen CB, et al. Thimerosal and the occurrence of autism: negative ecological evidence from Danish population-based data. *Pediatrics* 2003;112:604–6; Hviid A, Stellfeld M, Wohlfahrt J, et al. Association between thimerosal-containing vaccine and autism. *JAMA* 2003;290:1763–6.

54 Madsen KM, Hviid A, Vestergaard M, et al. A population-based study of measles, mumps, and rubella vaccination and autism.

55 Madsen KM, Lauritsen MB, Pedersen CB, et al. Thimerosal and the occurrence of autism: negative ecological evidence from Danish population-based data.

56 Hviid A, Stellfeld M, Wohlfahrt J, et al. Association between thimerosal-containing vaccine and autism.

57 Madsen KM, Hviid A, Vestergaard M, et al. A population-based study of measles, mumps, and rubella vaccination and autism.

58 DeStefano F, Bhasin TK, Thompson WW, et al. Age at first measles-mumps-rubella vaccination in children with autism and school-matched control subjects: a population-based study in metropolitan Atlanta.

59 Madsen KM, Lauritsen MB, Pedersen CB, et al. Thimerosal and the occurrence of autism: negative ecological evidence from Danish population-based data.

[60] Hviid A, Stellfeld M, Wohlfahrt J, et al. Association between thimerosal-containing vaccine and autism.

[61] Godlee F, Smith J, Marcovitch H. Wakefield's article linking MMR vaccine and autism was fraudulent.

[62] Ibid.

[63] Deer B. How the case against the MMR vaccine was fixed; Deer B. The Lancet's two days to bury bad news; Deer B. How the vaccine crisis was meant to make money; Deer B. Who saw the "histological findings"?; Deer B. Pathology reports solve "new bowel disease" riddle; Godlee F, Smith J, Marcovitch H. Wakefield's article linking MMR vaccine and autism was fraudulent; Godlee F. Institutional and editorial misconduct in the MMR scare; Deer B. Andrew Wakefield concocts a conspiracy.

[64] Miller S. Re: The unofficial vaccine educators: are CDC funded non-profits sufficiently independent? 2017; Nov. 18. https://www.bmj.com/content/359/bmj.j5104/rr-13.

[65] Physicians for Informed Consent. Measles – Vaccine Risk Statement (VRS). Oct. 2017. https://www.physiciansforinformedconsent.org/measles/vrs.

[66] Physicians for Informed Consent. Measles – Disease Information Statement (DIS). Oct. 2017. https://www.physiciansforinformedconsent.org/measles/dis.

[67] Vestergaard M, Hviid A, Madsen KM, et al. MMR vaccination and febrile seizures: evaluation of susceptible subgroups and long-term prognosis. *JAMA* 2004;292:351–357.

[68] Ibid.

[69] CDC. Measles. Undated. https://www.cdc.gov/vaccines/pubs/pinkbook/meas.html.

[70] Ibid.

[71] Physicians for Informed Consent. Measles – Vaccine Risk Statement (VRS).

[72] Ibid.

[73] Madsen KM, Hviid A, Vestergaard M, et al. A population-based study of measles, mumps, and rubella vaccination and autism.

[74] World Health Organization. Measles. 2018.

[75] Mina MJ, Metcalf CJ, de Swart RL, et al. Long-term measles-induced immunomodulation increases overall childhood infectious disease mortality. *Science* 2015;348:694–9.

[76] Aaby P, Benn CS. Developing the concept of beneficial nonspecific effect of live vaccines with epidemiological studies. *Clin Microbiol Infect* 2019;25:1459–67.

[77] Benn CS, Fisker AB, Rieckmann A, et al. How to evaluate potential non-specific effects of vaccines: The quest for randomized trials or time for triangulation? *Expert Rev Vaccines* 2018;17:411–20.

[78] World Health Organization. Measles. 2018; Nov. 29. https://www.who.int/en/news-room/fact-sheets/detail/measles.

[79] Huiming Y, Chaomin W, Meng M. Vitamin A for treating measles in children. *Cochrane Database Syst Rev* 2005;(4):CD001479.

[80] World Health Organization. Measles. 2018.

[81] Demicheli V, Rivetti A, Debalini MG, et al. Vaccines for measles, mumps and rubella in children. *Cochrane Database Syst Rev* 2012;(2):CD004407.

[82] CDC. Measles.

[83] Atkinson WL, Orenstein WA, Krugman S. The resurgence of measles in the United States, 1989–1990. *Annu Rev Med* 1992;43:451–63.

[84] Centers for Disease Control and Prevention. Complications of measles. 2019; Feb. 5. https://www.cdc.gov/measles/about/complications.html.

[85] Tanne JH. Measles: two US outbreaks are blamed on low vaccination rates. *BMJ* 2019;364:l312.

[86] Larsen K. Den desperate kamp mod mæslinger. *Ugeskr Læger* 2019; March 14.

[87] Osborne S. Measles outbreak kills 1,200 in Madagascar. *The Independent* 2019; Apr. 15.

[88] CDC. Measles.

CHAPTER 3

[1] Hope J. Why Japan banned MMR vaccine. *Daily Mail* 2019; May 13.

[2] Ibid.

[3] Dyer O. Philippines measles outbreak is deadliest yet as vaccine scepticism spurs disease comeback. *BMJ* 2019;364:l739.

[4] Olive JK, Hotez PJ, Damania A, et al. The state of the antivaccine movement in the United States: A focused examination of nonmedical exemptions in states and counties. *PLoS Med* 2018;15:e1002578.

[5] SB-277 Public health: vaccinations. 2015; June 30. http://leginfo.legislature.ca.gov /faces/billTextClient.xhtml?bill_id=201520160SB277.

[6] Delamater PL, Pingali SC, Buttenheim AM, et al. Elimination of nonmedical immunization exemptions in California and school-entry vaccine status. *Pediatrics* 2019;143(6).

[7] M-M-R* II. (MEASLES, MUMPS, and RUBELLA VIRUS VACCINE LIVE). https: //www.fda.gov/media/75191/download.

[8] Orenstein WA, Ahmed R. Simply put: Vaccination saves lives. *Proc Natl Acad Sci USA* 2017;114:4031–33.

[9] Tanne JH. Parents of US boy who survived tetanus after nearly $1m of care refuse vaccine. *BMJ* 2019;364:l1172.

[10] Finnegan G. Mandatory vaccination: does it work in Europe? *Vaccines Today* 2017; Nov. 27.

[11] Ibid.

[12] Doshi P. The unofficial vaccine educators: are CDC funded non-profits sufficiently independent? *BMJ* 2017;359:j5104.

[13] Gøtzsche PC. *Deadly medicines and organised crime: How big pharma has corrupted health care.* London: Radcliffe Publishing; 2013.

[14] Lacobucci G. NHS staff who refuse flu vaccine this winter will have to give reasons. *BMJ* 2017;359:j4766.

[15] Behrman A, Offley W. Should influenza vaccination be mandatory for healthcare workers? *BMJ* 2013;347:f6705.

[16] Ibid.

[17] McCartney M. New York University sacks professor for refusing flu shot. *BMJ* 2017;357:j1975.

[18] Siri & Glimstad LLP. Aaron Siri, attorney. https://www.sirillp.com/aaron-siri/.

[19] Finnegan G. Mandatory vaccination: does it work in Europe?

[20] Ibid.

[21] "Major interpellation for written answer with debate G-000010/2017," European Parliament, September 15, 2017. https://www.europarl.europa.eu/doceo/document/G -8-2017-000010_EN.html.

[22] Ibid.

[23] Siri & Glimstad LLP. Aaron Siri, attorney. https://www.sirillp.com/aaron-siri/.

[24] Gøtzsche PC. *Deadly psychiatry and organised denial.* Copenhagen: People's Press; 2015.

[25] Jefferson T. Scientist fires latest shot in mandatory flu vaccine debate. *Vancouver Sun* 2012; Nov. 19.

[26] Gøtzsche PC. *Deadly psychiatry and organised denial.*

[27] UNESCO, "Universal Declaration on Bioethics and Human Rights," October 19, 2005. http://portal.unesco.org/en/ev.php-URL_ID=31058&URL_DO=DO_TOPIC& URL_SECTION=201.html.

[28] Brewer NT, Chapman GB, Rothman AJ, et al. Increasing vaccination: putting psychological science into action. *Psychol Sci Public Interest* 2017;18:149–207.

CHAPTER 4

[1] Gøtzsche PC. *Survival in an overmedicated world: look up the evidence yourself.* Copenhagen: People's Press; 2019.

[2] Demicheli V, Jefferson T, Ferroni E, et al. Vaccines for preventing influenza in healthy adults. *Cochrane Database Syst Rev* 2018;2:CD001269.

[3] Jefferson T, Rivetti A, Di Pietrantonj C, et al. Vaccines for preventing influenza in healthy children. *Cochrane Database Syst Rev* 2018;2:CD004879.

[4] Ibid.

[5] Demicheli V, Jefferson T, Di Pietrantonj C, et al. Vaccines for preventing influenza in the elderly. *Cochrane Database Syst Rev* 2018;2:CD004876.

[6] Beyer WE, McElhaney J, Smith DJ, et al. Cochrane re-arranged: support for policies to vaccinate elderly people against influenza. *Vaccine* 2013;31:6030–3.

[7] Sørensen AM. Nyt studie slår fast: Ældre bør vaccineres mod influenza. *Videnskab dk* 2013; Oct. 28.

[8] Gøtzsche PC. *Death of a whistleblower and Cochrane's moral collapse.* Copenhagen: People's Press; 2019.

[9] Godlee F. Reinvigorating Cochrane. *BMJ* 2018;362:k3966.

[10] https://www.viroclinics.com/.

[11] Fireman B, Lee J, Lewis N, et al. Influenza vaccination and mortality: differentiating vaccine effects from bias. *Am J Epidemiol* 2009;170:650–6.

[12] Ibid.

[13] Ibid.

[14] https://www.fda.gov/vaccines-blood-biologics/vaccines/influenza-virus-vaccine -quadrivalent-types-and-types-b.

[15] Demicheli V, Jefferson T, Ferroni E, et al. Vaccines for preventing influenza in healthy adults.

[16] Gigerenzer G. *Risk savvy. How to make good decisions.* New York: Penguin Group; 2014, page 210.

[17] Gøtzsche PC, Jørgensen KJ. Screening for breast cancer with mammography. *Cochrane Database Syst Rev* 2013;6:CD001877.

[18] Jefferson T, Jones M, Doshi P, et al. Oseltamivir for influenza in adults and children: systematic review of clinical study reports and summary of regulatory comments. *BMJ* 2014;348:g2545.

[19] Ibid.

20 Gøtzsche PC. *Deadly medicines and organised crime: How big pharma has corrupted health care*. London: Radcliffe Publishing; 2013.

21 Ibid.

22 Gøtzsche PC. *Survival in an overmedicated world: look up the evidence yourself.*

23 Pedante I, Dal Monte PP. Immunità di legge. *I vaccini obbligatori tra scienza al governo e governo della scienza*. Bologna: Ariana Editrice; 2018.

24 Ibid.

25 Epstein H. Flu warning: Beware the drug companies! *New York Review of Books* 2011; May 12.

26 Ibid.

27 Ibid.

28 Lenzer J. Centers for Disease Control and Prevention: protecting the private good? *BMJ* 2015;350:h2362.

29 Jefferson T, Jones M, Doshi P, et al. Oseltamivir for influenza in adults and children: systematic review of clinical study reports and summary of regulatory comments. *BMJ* 2014;348:g2545.

30 https://www.fda.gov/vaccines-blood-biologics/vaccines/influenza-virus-vaccine -quadrivalent-types-and-types-b.

31 Demicheli V, Jefferson T, Ferroni E, et al. Vaccines for preventing influenza in healthy adults.

32 Centers for Disease Control and Prevention. Vaccine effectiveness: How well do the flu vaccines work? 2018; 12 Oct. https://www.cdc.gov/flu/vaccines-work/vaccineeffect .htm.

33 Centers for Disease Control and Prevention. Influenza vaccination information for health care workers. 2018; Nov. 16. https://www.cdc.gov/flu/professionals/healthcareworkers .htm.

34 Ahmed F, Lindley M, Allred N, et al. Effect of influenza vaccination of healthcare personnel on morbidity and mortality among patients: systematic review and grading of evidence. *Clin Infect Dis* 2014;58:50–7; Griffin MR. Influenza vaccination of healthcare workers: making the grade for action. *Clin Infect Diseases* 2014;58:58–60.

35 Fireman B, Lee J, Lewis N, et al. Influenza vaccination and mortality: differentiating vaccine effects from bias.

36 Thomas RE, Jefferson T, Lasserson TJ. Influenza vaccination for healthcare workers who care for people aged 60 or older living in long-term care institutions. *Cochrane Database Syst Rev* 2016;6:CD005187.

37 Gøtzsche PC. *Mammography screening: truth, lies and controversy*. London: Radcliffe Publishing; 2012.

38 Thomas RE, Jefferson T, Lasserson TJ. Influenza vaccination for healthcare workers who care for people aged 60 or older living in long-term care institutions.

39 Griffin MR. Influenza vaccination of healthcare workers: making the grade for action.

40 McCartney M. New York University sacks professor for refusing flu shot. *BMJ* 2017;357:j1975.

41 Ibid.

42 Centers for Disease Control and Prevention. Influenza vaccination information for health care workers.

43 Vainio H, Bianchini F. Breast Cancer Screening. *IARC Handbooks of Cancer Prevention*, Vol 7. Lyon, France: IARC Press; 2002.

44 Janzon L, Andersson I. The Malmö mammographic screening trial. In: *Cancer Screening*, Miller AB, Chamberlain J, Day NE, et al. (eds). Cambridge: Cambridge University Press; 1991.

45 Centers for Disease Control and Prevention. Vaccine effectiveness: How well do the flu vaccines work?

46 Gøtzsche PC. *Deadly psychiatry and organised denial*. Copenhagen: People's Press; 2015.

47 Centers for Disease Control and Prevention, "What are the benefits of flu vaccination?" https://www.cdc.gov/flu/prevent/vaccine-benefits.htm.

48 Ferdinands JM, Olsho LE, Agan AA, et al. Effectiveness of influenza vaccine against life-threatening RT-PCR-confirmed influenza illness in US children, 2010–2012. *J Infect Dis* 2014;210:674–83.

49 Ibid.

50 Deeks JJ, Dinnes J, D'Amico R, et al. Evaluating non-randomised intervention studies. *Health Technol Assess* 2003;7:1–173.

51 Rondy M, El Omeiri N, Thompson MG, et al. Effectiveness of influenza vaccines in preventing severe influenza illness among adults: a systematic review and meta-analysis of test-negative design case-control studies. *J Infect* 2017;75:381–94.

52 Thompson MG, Pierse N, Sue Huang Q, et al. Influenza vaccine effectiveness in preventing influenza-associated intensive care admissions and attenuating severe disease among adults in New Zealand 2012–2015. *Vaccine* 2018;36:5916–25.

53 Ferdinands JM, Olsho LE, Agan AA, et al. Effectiveness of influenza vaccine against life-threatening RT-PCR-confirmed influenza illness in US children.

54 Ferdinands JM, Olsho LE, Agan AA, et al. Effectiveness of influenza vaccine against life-threatening RT-PCR-confirmed influenza illness in US children; Rondy M, El Omeiri N, Thompson MG, et al. Effectiveness of influenza vaccines in preventing severe influenza illness among adults: a systematic review and meta-analysis of test-negative design case-control studies; Thompson MG, Pierse N, Sue Huang Q, et al. Influenza vaccine effectiveness in preventing influenza-associated intensive care admissions and attenuating severe disease among adults in New Zealand 2012–2015.

55 Centers for Disease Control and Prevention. Vaccine effectiveness: How well do the flu vaccines work?

56 Flannery B, Reynolds SB, Blanton L, et al. Influenza vaccine effectiveness against pediatric deaths: 2010–2014. *Pediatrics* 2017;139:e20164244.

57 Centers for Disease Control and Prevention. Vaccine effectiveness: How well do the flu vaccines work?

58 Ibid.

59 Casado I, Dominguez A, Toledo D, et al. Repeated influenza vaccination for preventing severe and fatal influenza infection in older adults: a multicentre case-control study. *CMAJ* 2018;190:E3–12.

60 Crowe K. Flu deaths reality check. Credibility of flu models disputed. CBC News 2012; Nov. 25.

61 Ibid.

62 Ibid.

63 Nordmændene kan noget, som danskerne ikke kan - kun én procent af de unge kvinder ryger. TV2 Nyheder 2018; Aug. 7.

64 Crowe K. Flu deaths reality check. Credibility of flu models disputed. CBC News.

65 Krogsbøll LT, Jørgensen KJ, Gøtzsche PC. General health checks in adults for reducing morbidity and mortality from disease. *Cochrane Database Syst Rev* 2019;1:CD009009.

66 Gøtzsche PC. *Survival in an overmedicated world: look up the evidence yourself.*

67 Gøtzsche PC. "I don't want the truth, I want something I can tell Parliament!" *BMJ* 2013;347:f5222.

68 Ibid.

69 Centers for Disease Control and Prevention. Vaccine effectiveness: How well do the flu vaccines work?

70 Thompson MG, Pierse N, Sue Huang Q, et al. Influenza vaccine effectiveness in preventing influenza-associated intensive care admissions and attenuating severe disease among adults in New Zealand 2012–2015.

71 Madhi SA, Cutland CL, Kuwanda L, et al. Influenza vaccination of pregnant women and protection of their infants. *N Engl J Med* 2014;371:918–31.

72 Salam RA, Das JK, Dojo Soeandy C, et al. Impact of Haemophilus influenzae type B (Hib) and viral influenza vaccinations in pregnancy for improving maternal, neonatal and infant health outcomes. *Cochrane Database Syst Rev* 2015;6:CD009982.

73 Donzelli A. Influenza vaccination for all pregnant women? So far the less biased evidence does not favour it. *Hum Vaccin Immunother* 2019;Jan. 11:1–6.

74 Steinhoff MC, Katz J, Englund J, et al. Year-round influenza immunisation during pregnancy in Nepal: a phase 4, randomised, placebo-controlled trial. *Lancet Infect Dis* 2017;17:981–9.

75 Centers for Disease Control and Prevention. Vaccine effectiveness: How well do the flu vaccines work?

76 Tapia MD, Sow SO, Tamboura B, et al. Maternal immunisation with trivalent inactivated influenza vaccine for prevention of influenza in infants in Mali: a prospective, active-controlled, observer-blind, randomised phase 4 trial. *Lancet Infect Dis* 2016;16:1026–35.

77 Centers for Disease Control and Prevention. Vaccine effectiveness: How well do the flu vaccines work?; Centers for Disease Control and Prevention. Influenza vaccination information for health care workers.

78 Centers for Disease Control and Prevention. Influenza vaccination information for health care workers.

79 https://www.fda.gov/vaccines-blood-biologics/vaccines/influenza-virus-vaccine-quadrivalent-types-and-types-b.

80 Centers for Disease Control and Prevention. Influenza (Flu) Vaccine Safety. https://www.cdc.gov/flu/prevent/vaccinesafety.htm.

81 Madhi SA, Cutland CL, Kuwanda L, et al. Influenza vaccination of pregnant women and protection of their infants.

82 Lundh A, Barbateskovic M, Hróbjartsson A, et al. Conflicts of interest at medical journals: the influence of industry-supported randomised trials on journal impact factors and revenue – cohort study. *PLoS Med* 2010;7:e1000354.

83 Gøtzsche PC. *Deadly medicines and organised crime: How big pharma has corrupted health care.*

84 Ibid.

85 Madhi SA, Cutland CL, Kuwanda L, et al. Influenza vaccination of pregnant women and protection of their infants. *N Engl J Med* 2014;371:918–31.

86 Centers for Disease Control and Prevention. Influenza (Flu) Vaccine Safety.

87 Gøtzsche PC. *Deadly medicines and organised crime: How big pharma has corrupted health care*; Gøtzsche PC. *Deadly psychiatry and organised denial.*

88 Institutet för Hälsa och Välfärd. Förhöjd narkolepsirisk i två år efter Pandemrix-vaccinationen. 2014; June; Nohynek H, Jokinen J, Partinen M, et al. AS03 adjuvanted AH1N1 vaccine associated with an abrupt increase in the incidence of childhood narcolepsy in Finland. *PLoS One* 2012;7:e33536.

89 Vogel G. Why a pandemic flu shot caused narcolepsy. Science 2015; July 1.

90 Demicheli V, Jefferson T, Ferroni E, et al. Vaccines for preventing influenza in healthy adults; Jefferson T, Rivetti A, Di Pietrantonj C, et al. Vaccines for preventing influenza in healthy children; Demicheli V, Jefferson T, Di Pietrantonj C, et al. Vaccines for preventing influenza in the elderly.

91 Jefferson T, Rivetti A, Di Pietrantonj C, et al. Vaccines for preventing influenza in healthy children; Doshi P. Influenza vaccines: Time for a rethink. *JAMA Intern Med* 2013;173:1014–6.

92 Doshi P. Influenza vaccines: Time for a rethink.

93 Skowronski DM, De Serres G, Crowcroft NS, et al. Association between the 2008–09 seasonal influenza vaccine and pandemic H1N1 illness during spring–summer 2009: four observational studies from Canada. *PLoS Med* 2010;7:e1000258.

94 Doshi P. Influenza vaccines: Time for a rethink.

95 Centers for Disease Control and Prevention. Vaccine effectiveness: How well do the flu vaccines work?

96 Vogel G. Why a pandemic flu shot caused narcolepsy; Doshi P. Influenza vaccines: Time for a rethink; Skowronski DM, De Serres G, Crowcroft NS, et al. Association between the 2008–09 seasonal influenza vaccine and pandemic H1N1 illness during spring–summer 2009: four observational studies from Canada; Benn CS, Fisker AB, Aaby P (eds.). Bandim Health Project, 1978–2018. Forty years of contradicting conventional wisdom. Contact: bandim@ssi.dk. All publications are available at https://www.bandim.org/publications.aspx.

97 Centers for Disease Control and Prevention. Influenza (Flu) Vaccine Safety.

98 Centers for Disease Control and Prevention. Vaccine effectiveness: How well do the flu vaccines work?; Skowronski DM, De Serres G, Crowcroft NS, et al. Association between the 2008–09 seasonal influenza vaccine and pandemic H1N1 illness during spring–summer 2009: four observational studies from Canada.

99 CDC. Early-Season Flu Vaccination Coverage – United States, Nov. 2018. https://www.cdc.gov/flu/fluvaxview/nifs-estimates-nov2018.htm; Statens Serum Institut. Andel vaccineret med sæsoninfluenza-vaccination (aldersgruppe), Sæson: 2009/2010–2018/2019. https://statistik.ssi.dk//sygdomsdata#!/?vaccination=14&sex=3&agegroup=10&landsdel=100&xaxis=AgeGroup&yaxis=Total&show=Table&datatype=Vaccination.

100 WHO. Influenza, vaccine use. https://www.who.int/influenza/vaccines/use/en/.

101 Benn CS, Fisker AB, Aaby P (eds.). Bandim Health Project, 1978–2018. Forty years of contradicting conventional wisdom.

102 Jefferson T, Rivetti A, Di Pietrantonj C, et al. Vaccines for preventing influenza in healthy children.

103 Demicheli V, Jefferson T, Di Pietrantonj C, et al. Vaccines for preventing influenza in the elderly.

104 Jørgensen KJ, Gøtzsche PC. Who evaluates public health programmes? A review of the NHS Breast Screening Programme. *J R Soc Med* 2010;103:14–20.

105 Centers for Disease Control and Prevention. Vaccine effectiveness: How well do the flu vaccines work?

[106] Gøtzsche PC. Survival in an overmedicated world: look up the evidence yourself.

[107] Evans SS, Repasky EA, Fisher DT. Fever and the thermal regulation of immunity: the immune system feels the heat. *Nat Rev Immunol* 2015;15:335–49.

CHAPTER 5

[1] Severe acute respiratory syndrome. https://en.wikipedia.org/wiki/Severe_acute_respiratory_syndrome.

[2] European Centre for Disease Prevention and Control. MERS-CoV worldwide overview. https://www.ecdc.europa.eu/en/middle-east-respiratory-syndrome-coronavirus-mers-cov-situation-update.

[3] Readfern G. How did coronavirus start and where did it come from? Was it really Wuhan's animal market? *The Guardian* 2020; Apr. 9.

[4] Davidson H. Chinese inquiry exonerates Coronavirus whistleblower doctor. *The Guardian* 2020; Mar. 20.

[5] Ibid.

[6] Riordan P, Manson K, Hille K, Cookson C. Taiwan says WHO failed to act on coronavirus transmission warning. *Financial Times* 2020; Mar. 20.

[7] Davidson H. Chinese inquiry exonerates Coronavirus whistleblower doctor.

[8] Covid: WHO team investigating virus origins denied entry to China. BBC News 2021; Jan. 6.

[9] Gøtzsche PC. Covid-19: Are we the victims of mass panic? *BMJ* 2020; Mar. 8. https://www.bmj.com/content/368/bmj.m800/rr-1; Gøtzsche PC. The Coronavirus mass panic is not justified. *Deadly Medicines* 2020; Mar. 24. https://www.deadlymedicines.dk/the-coronavirus-mass-panic-is-not-justified/.

[10] Jefferson T, Del Mar CB, Dooley L, Ferroni E, Al-Ansary LA, Bawazeer GA, et al. Physical interventions to interrupt or reduce the spread of respiratory viruses. *Cochrane Database Syst Rev* 2020;11:CD006207.

[11] Gøtzsche PC. Corona update: I have lost confidence in the authorities. *Institute for Scientific Freedom* 2020; Nov. 12. https://www.scientificfreedom.dk/2020/11/12/corona-update-i-have-lost-confidence-in-the-authorities/.

[12] Chu DK, Akl EA, Duda S, Solo K, Yaacoub S, Schünemann HJ, et al. Physical distancing, face masks, and eye protection to prevent person-to-person transmission of SARS-CoV-2 and COVID-19: a systematic review and meta-analysis. *Lancet* 2020;395:1973–87.

[13] Heneghan C, Jefferson T. COVID-19: Evidence is lacking for 2 meter distancing. Centre for Evidence-Based Medicine 2020; June 19.

[14] Bundgaard H, Bundgaard JS, Raaschou-Pedersen DET, von Buchwald C, Todsen T, Norsk JB, et al. Effectiveness of adding a mask recommendation to other public health measures to prevent SARS-CoV-2 infection in Danish mask wearers: a randomized controlled trial. *Ann Intern Med* 2020; Nov. 18: M20-6817. doi: 10.7326/M20-6817. Epub ahead of print. PMID: 33205991; PMCID: PMC7707213.

[15] Boccia S, Ricciardi W, Ioannidis JPA. What other countries can learn from Italy during the COVID-19 pandemic. *JAMA Intern Med* 2020; Apr. 7. doi: 10.1001/jamainternmed.2020.1447. [Epub ahead of print.]

[16] Jefferson T, Del Mar CB, Dooley L, Ferroni E, Al-Ansary LA, Bawazeer GA, et al. Physical interventions to interrupt or reduce the spread of respiratory viruses.

[17] COVID curve tracker (regularly updated). https://covidcurvetracker.org/.

[18] Møller AS. Ny hastelov på vej: Regeringen vil forbyde forsamlinger på over to personer. TV2 2020: Mar. 25.

[19] Gordon J. Wear a mask while having sex, Canada's top doctor suggests. MSN 2020; Sept. 2.

[20] Viner RM, Russell SJ, Croker H, Packer J, Ward J, Stansfield C, et al. School closure and management practices during coronavirus outbreaks including COVID-19: a rapid systematic review. *Lancet Child Adolesc Health* 2020; Apr. 6. pii: S2352-4642(20)30095-X. doi: 10.1016/S2352-4642(20)30095-X. [Epub ahead of print.]

[21] Average age of death (median and mean) of persons whose death was due to COVID-19 or involved COVID-19, by sex, deaths registered up to week ending Oct. 2, 2020, England and Wales. 2020; 14 Oct. https://www.ons.gov.uk/.

[22] Jamison P. A top scientist questioned virus lockdowns on Fox News. The backlash was fierce. *Washington Post* 2020; Dec. 16.

[23] European Centre for Disease Prevention and Control and European Union Aviation Safety Agency. Guidelines for COVID-19 testing and quarantine of air travellers – Addendum to the Aviation Health Safety Protocol. 2020; Dec. 2.

[24] Bourke L. 'A bit premature': Global airline body pours cold water on Qantas' no vaccine, no fly stance. *Sydney Morning Herald* 2020; Nov. 25.

[25] Jefferson T, Del Mar CB, Dooley L, Ferroni E, Al-Ansary LA, Bawazeer GA, et al. Physical interventions to interrupt or reduce the spread of respiratory viruses.

[26] Schmidt AL, Rasmussen LI. Verdensberømt dansk professor: "Det, Danmark gør lige nu, er en isolationsstrategi med et naivt håb om, at virus forsvinder og aldrig kommer igen." *Politiken* 2020; Mar. 29.

[27] Jefferson T, Del Mar CB, Dooley L, Ferroni E, Al-Ansary LA, Bawazeer GA, et al. Physical interventions to interrupt or reduce the spread of respiratory viruses.

[28] Ioannidis JPA. A fiasco in the making? As the coronavirus pandemic takes hold, we are making decisions without reliable data. 2020; Mar. 17. https://www.statnews.com/.

[29] Ibid.

[30] Nisgaard A. 23 millioner indbyggere og kun syv døde: Derfor har Taiwan så godt styr på corona Mens Danmark lukker ned, går taiwanerne til koncert og på natklub. DR Nyheder 2020; Dec. 19.

[31] Ibid.

[32] COVID-19 Coronavirus pandemic. https://www.worldometers.info/coronavirus/. Accessed Dec. 20, 2020.

[33] Ibid.

[34] Ibid.

[35] https://www.euromomo.eu/graphs-and-maps. Accessed Dec. 29, 2020.

[36] Berg T, Lundbye AB. Statsminister advarer om coronavirus - arrangementer med over 1000 mennesker bør aflyses. TV2 2020; Mar. 6.

[37] Juncker SH. Mens Danmark lukker ned, fortsætter hverdagen i Sverige: Hvorfor reagerer de to lande så forskelligt? Information 2020; Mar. 14.

[38] Jørgensen AS, Mansø RG, Tofte LR. Forsamlinger og aktiviteter med mere end 10 personer bliver forbudt. DR 2020; Mar. 17.

[39] Leonhardt D, Leatherby L. Where the virus is growing most: countries with "illiberal populist" leaders. *New York Times* 2020; June 10.

[40] Jamison P. A top scientist questioned virus lockdowns on Fox News. The backlash was fierce. *Washington Post* 2020; Dec. 16.

41 Leonhardt D, Leatherby L. Where the virus is growing most: countries with "illiberal populist" leaders.

42 Yamey G, Wenham C. The U.S. and U.K. were the two best prepared nations to tackle a pandemic - what went wrong? *Time* 2020; July 1.

43 Coronavirus: Outcry after Trump suggests injecting disinfectant as treatment. BBC News 2020; Apr. 24.

44 Kristensen TK. Drop selvfedheden: Danmark er ikke verdensmester i coronakamp. Politiken 2020; July 4.

45 Yamey G, Wenham C. The U.S. and U.K. were the two best prepared nations to tackle a pandemic - what went wrong?

46 Ibid.

47 Godlee F. Covid-19: We need new thinking and new leadership. *BMJ* 2020;371:m4358.

48 Leonhardt D, Leatherby L. Where the virus is growing most: countries with "illiberal populist" leaders.

49 Panum PL. Observations made during the epidemic of measles on the Faroe Islands in the year 1846. http://www.med.mcgill.ca/epidemiology/courses/EPIB591/Fall%20-2010/mid-term%20presentations/Paper9.pdf.

50 WHO Director-General's opening remarks at the media briefing on COVID-19. World Health Organization 2020; Mar. 3. https://www.who.int/.

51 Mallapaty S. What the cruise-ship outbreaks reveal about COVID-19. *Nature* 2020; Mar. 26; Ginn A. 2020; Mar. 20 (regularly updated). https://docs.google.com/document/d/1EC7mTsuBAScE_yrgZz26DevuZJHbtDbbvGgf2WRlEJc/edit#.

52 Mallapaty S. What the cruise-ship outbreaks reveal about COVID-19.

53 WHO Director-General's opening remarks at the media briefing on COVID-19. World Health Organization.

54 Ioannidis JPA. A fiasco in the making? As the coronavirus pandemic takes hold, we are making decisions without reliable data.

55 Jørgensen AS. Dødelighed skal formentlig tælles i promiller: Danske blodprøver kaster nyt lys over coronasmitten. DR TV 2020; Apr. 8.

56 Ioannidis JPA. A fiasco in the making? As the coronavirus pandemic takes hold, we are making decisions without reliable data; Mallapaty S. What the cruise-ship outbreaks reveal about COVID-19.

57 Ioannidis JPA. A fiasco in the making? As the coronavirus pandemic takes hold, we are making decisions without reliable data.

58 Ioannidis JPA. Infection fatality rate of COVID-19. *Bull World Health Organ* 2021 (in press).

59 Wong JY, Kelly H, Ip DK, Wu JT, Leung GM, Cowling BJ. Case fatality risk of influenza A (H1N1pdm09): a systematic review. *Epidemiology* 2013;24:830–41.

60 Boccia S, Ricciardi W, Ioannidis JPA. What other countries can learn from Italy during the COVID-19 pandemic. *JAMA Intern Med* 2020; Apr. 7. doi: 10.1001/jamainternmed.2020.1447. [Epub ahead of print.]

61 Meduri GU, Siemieniuk RAC, Ness RA, Seyler SJ. Prolonged low-dose methylprednisolone treatment is highly effective in reducing duration of mechanical ventilation and mortality in patients with ARDS. *J Intensive Care* 2018;6:53.

62 WHO Solidarity trial consortium. Repurposed antiviral drugs for COVID-19 interim WHO SOLIDARITY trial results. 2020; Oct. 15. https://www.medrxiv.org/content/10.1101/2020.10.15.20209817v1.full.pdf.

[63] Lenzer J, Brownlee S. Pandemic science out of control. *Issues in Science and Technology* 2020; Apr. 28.

[64] Rowland C. Government researchers changed metric to measure coronavirus drug remdesivir during clinical trial. *Washington Post* 2020; May 2.

[65] Lenzer J, Brownlee S. Pandemic science out of control.

[66] US antidepressant fills increased 20%; HCQ rose 525%. *The Pharma Letter* 2020; Dec. 19.

[67] WHO Solidarity trial consortium. Repurposed antiviral drugs for COVID-19 interim WHO SOLIDARITY trial results. 2020; 15 Oct. https://www.medrxiv.org/content/10.1101/2020.10.15.20209817v1.full.pdf.

[68] Rowland C. Government researchers changed metric to measure coronavirus drug remdesivir during clinical trial.

[69] Beigel JH, Tomashek KM, Dodd LE, Mehta AK, Zingman BS, Kalil AC, et al. Remdesivir for the treatment of Covid-19 - preliminary report. *N Engl J Med* 2020; May 20. https://www.nejm.org/doi/pdf/10.1056/NEJMoa2007764.

[70] Gøtzsche PC. Remdesivir against coronavirus, hope or hype? *Institute for Scientific Freedom* 2020; June 1. https://www.scientificfreedom.dk/2020/06/01/remdesivir-against -coronavirus-hope-or-hype/.

[71] Gøtzsche PC. *Deadly medicines and organised crime: How big pharma has corrupted health care*. London: Radcliffe Publishing; 2013.

[72] WHO Solidarity trial consortium. Repurposed antiviral drugs for COVID-19 interim WHO SOLIDARITY trial results.

[73] Ibid.

[74] Wang Y, Zhang D, Du G, Du R, Zhao J, Jin Y, et al. Remdesivir in adults with severe COVID-19: a randomised, double-blind, placebo-controlled, multicentre trial. *Lancet* 2020;395:1569–78.

[75] Cohen J, Kupferschmidt K. The "very, very bad look" of remdesivir, the first FDA-approved COVID-19 drug. *Science* 2020; Oct. 27.

[76] Liu A. COVID-19 fighter remdesivir racks up $873M as Gilead plays defense on unflattering WHO data. 2020; Oct. 29. https://www.fiercepharma.com/marketing /remdesivir-sales-hit-873m-as-gilead-gets-defensive-against-who-data-covid-19-drug.

[77] European Medicines Agency. Update on remdesivir - EMA will evaluate new data from Solidarity trial. 2020; 20 Nov. https://www.ema.europa.eu/en/news/update-remdesivir -ema-will-evaluate-new-data-solidarity-trial.

[78] Voysey M, Clemens SAC, Madhi SA, Weckx LY, Folegatti PM, Aley PK, et al. Safety and efficacy of the ChAdOx1 nCoV-19 vaccine (AZD1222) against SARS-CoV-2: an interim analysis of four randomised controlled trials in Brazil, South Africa, and the UK. *Lancet* 2020; Dec. 8: S0140-6736(20)32661-1. doi: 10.1016/S0140-6736(20)32661-1. (Epub ahead of print.) PMID: 33306989; PMCID: PMC7723445.

[79] Polack FP, Thomas SJ, Kitchin N, Absalon J, Gurtman A, Lockhart S, et al. Safety and efficacy of the BNT162b2 mRNA Covid-19 Vaccine. *N Engl J Med* 2020;383:2603–15; Baden LR, El Sahly HM, Essink B, Kotloff K, Frey S, Novak S, et al. Efficacy and safety of the mRNA-1273 SARS-CoV-2 vaccine. *N Engl J Med* 2020; 30 Dec. DOI: 10.1056/ NEJMe2035557.

[80] Voysey M, Clemens SAC, Madhi SA, Weckx LY, Folegatti PM, Aley PK, et al. Safety and efficacy of the ChAdOx1 nCoV-19 vaccine (AZD1222) against SARS-CoV-2: an interim analysis of four randomised controlled trials in Brazil, South Africa, and the UK.

81 Polack FP, Thomas SJ, Kitchin N, Absalon J, Gurtman A, Lockhart S, et al. Safety and
    efficacy of the BNT162b2 mRNA Covid-19 Vaccine.

82 FDA briefing document. Pfizer-BioNTech COVID-19 vaccine. 2020; Dec. 10. https:
    //www.fda.gov/media/144245/download.

83 Voysey M, Clemens SAC, Madhi SA, Weckx LY, Folegatti PM, Aley PK, et al. Safety
    and efficacy of the ChAdOx1 nCoV-19 vaccine (AZD1222) against SARS-CoV-2: an
    interim analysis of four randomised controlled trials in Brazil, South Africa, and the UK.

84 Polack FP, Thomas SJ, Kitchin N, Absalon J, Gurtman A, Lockhart S, et al. Safety and
    efficacy of the BNT162b2 mRNA Covid-19 Vaccine.

85 Baden LR, El Sahly HM, Essink B, Kotloff K, Frey S, Novak S, et al, Efficacy and safety
    of the mRNA-1273 SARS-CoV-2 vaccine.

86 Voysey M, Clemens SAC, Madhi SA, Weckx LY, Folegatti PM, Aley PK, et al. Safety
    and efficacy of the ChAdOx1 nCoV-19 vaccine (AZD1222) against SARS-CoV-2: an
    interim analysis of four randomised controlled trials in Brazil, South Africa, and the UK.

87 Polack FP, Thomas SJ, Kitchin N, Absalon J, Gurtman A, Lockhart S, et al. Safety and
    efficacy of the BNT162b2 mRNA Covid-19 Vaccine.

88 FDA briefing document. Pfizer-BioNTech COVID-19 vaccine.

89 Polack FP, Thomas SJ, Kitchin N, Absalon J, Gurtman A, Lockhart S, et al. Safety and
    efficacy of the BNT162b2 mRNA Covid-19 Vaccine.

90 FDA briefing document. Pfizer-BioNTech COVID-19 vaccine.

91 Ibid.

92 Ibid.

93 Baden LR, El Sahly HM, Essink B, Kotloff K, Frey S, Novak S, et al, Efficacy and safety
    of the mRNA-1273 SARS-CoV-2 vaccine.

94 Polack FP, Thomas SJ, Kitchin N, Absalon J, Gurtman A, Lockhart S, et al. Safety and
    efficacy of the BNT162b2 mRNA Covid-19 Vaccine.

95 Voysey M, Clemens SAC, Madhi SA, Weckx LY, Folegatti PM, Aley PK, et al. Safety
    and efficacy of the ChAdOx1 nCoV-19 vaccine (AZD1222) against SARS-CoV-2: an
    interim analysis of four randomised controlled trials in Brazil, South Africa, and the UK.

96 Ibid.

97 Demasi M. Elation or caution over COVID-19 vaccines? The evidence so far. Institute
    for Scientific Freedom 2020; Dec. 11. https://www.scientificfreedom.dk/2020/12/11
    /elation-or-caution-over-covid-19-vaccines-the-evidence-so-far/.

98 The Gamaleya National Centre. The first interim data analysis of the Sputnik V vaccine
    against COVID-19 phase III clinical trials in the Russian Federation demonstrated
    92% efficacy. 2020; Nov. 11. https://sputnikvaccine.com/newsroom/pressreleases/the
    -first-interim-data-analysis-of-the-sputnik-v-vaccine-against-covid-19-phase-iii-clinical
    -trials-/.

99 Doshi P. Will covid-19 vaccines save lives? Current trials aren't designed to tell us. *BMJ*
    2020;371:m4037.

100 Ibid.

101 Dyer O. White House demands to know how UK approved vaccine before FDA. *BMJ*
    2020;371:m4725.

102 Schmidt AL, Rasmussen LI. Verdensberømt dansk professor: "Det, Danmark gør lige
    nu, er en isolationsstrategi med et naivt håb om, at virus forsvinder og aldrig kommer
    igen." *Politiken* 2020; Mar. 29.

103 Demasi M. Elation or caution over COVID-19 vaccines? The evidence so far.

[104] Chadwick L, Monella LM. Which parts of Europe are likely to be most hesitant about a COVID-19 vaccine? 2020; Dec. 9. https://www.euronews.com/.

[105] Lumley SF, Wei J, O'Donnell D, Stoesser NE, Matthews PC, Howarth A, et al. The duration, dynamics and determinants of SARS-CoV-2 antibody responses in individual healthcare workers. 2020; Nov. 4. https://doi.org/10.1101/2020.11.02.20224824.

[106] Choi KR. A nursing researcher's experience in a COVID-19 vaccine trial. *JAMA Intern Med* 2020; Dec. 7. doi:10.1001/jamainternmed.2020.7087.

[107] American Academy of Family Physicians. COVID-19 vaccine FAQ. 2020; Dec. 17 (or later). https://www.aafp.org/dam/AAFP/documents/patient_care/public_health /COVID19-Vaccine-FAQs.pdf.

[108] Benn CS, Aaby P. Vaccineforskere Benn og Aaby: Skal vi vaccinere børn mod COVID-19, når muligheden kommer? *Ræson* 2020; Nov. 11.

[109] Ibid.

[110] Ibid.

[111] Demasi M. Elation or caution over COVID-19 vaccines? The evidence so far. Institute for Scientific Freedom 2020; 11 Dec. https://www.scientificfreedom.dk/2020/12/11 /elation-or-caution-over-covid-19-vaccines-the-evidence-so-far/.

[112] Statens Serum Institut. Dødsfald per aldersgruppe. https://experience.arcgis.com /experience/aa41b29149f24e20a4007a0c4e13db1d. Accessed Jan. 1, 2021.

[113] Danmarks Statistik. Døde efter køn, alder og dødsårsag. https://www.statbank.dk /statbank5a/SelectVarVal/Define.asp?Maintable=DOD1&PLanguage=0. Accessed Jan. 1, 2021.

[114] O'Driscoll M, Ribeiro Dos Santos G, Wang L, Cummings DAT, Azman AS, Paireau J, et al. Age-specific mortality and immunity patterns of SARS-CoV-2. *Nature* 2020; Nov. 2. doi: 10.1038/s41586-020-2918-0. (Epub ahead of print.) PMID: 33137809.

[115] Weekly updates by select demographic and geographic characteristics. Provisional death counts for Coronavirus Disease 2019 (COVID-19). https://www.cdc.gov/nchs/nvss /vsrr/covid_weekly/index.htm#AgeAndSex.

[116] WHO Director General's opening remarks at the media briefing on COVID-19. World Health Organization 2020; Mar. 3. https://www.who.int/.

[117] Thacker P. Conflicts of interest among the UK government's covid-19 advisers. *BMJ* 2020;371:m4716.

[118] Abbassi K. Covid-19: politicisation, "corruption," and suppression of science. *BMJ* 2020;371:m4425.

[119] Thacker P. Conflicts of interest among the UK government's covid-19 advisers.

[120] Roach A. Matt Hancock denies conflict of interest in Patrick Vallance holding vaccine company shares. *Evening Standard* 2020; Sept. 24.

[121] Braithwaite T. Why the Pfizer CEO selling 62% of his stock the same day as the vaccine announcement looks bad. *Financial Times* 2020; Nov. 13.

[122] Møller P. Minister kom til at afsløre hemmelig prisliste - så meget koster de forskellige vacciner. TV2 Nyheder 2020; Dec. 19.

[123] Ibid.

[124] Yan BW, Sloan FA, Dudley RA. How influenza vaccination rate variation could inform pandemic-era vaccination efforts. *J Gen Intern Med* 2020;35:3401–3.

[125] UNESCO. Universal Declaration on Bioethics and Human Rights. 2005; Oct. 19. http: //portal.unesco.org/en/ev.php-URL_ID=31058&URL_DO=DO_TOPIC&URL _SECTION=201.html.

[126] Wehenkel C. Positive association between COVID-19 deaths and influenza vaccination rates in elderly people worldwide. *PeerJ* 2020;8:e10112 DOI 10.7717/peerj.l0112.

[127] Zein JG, Whelan G, Erzurum SC. Safety of influenza vaccine during COVID-19. *J Clin Transl Sci* 2020 (in press). 10.1017/cts.2020.543.

[128] Cookson C. UK to test vaccines on volunteers deliberately infected with Covid-19. *Financial Times* 2020; Sept. 23.

[129] Ioannidis JPA. A fiasco in the making? As the coronavirus pandemic takes hold, we are making decisions without reliable data.

[130] Cookson C. UK to test vaccines on volunteers deliberately infected with Covid-19.

[131] Orry F, Bech TH, Olsgaard G. Eksperter efter ny SSI-rapport: Intet tyder på, at omdiskuteret virusvariant udfordrer vacciner. DR Nyheder 2020; 11 Nov.

[132] Gøtzsche PC. The coronavirus has created a nanny state. Institute for Scientific Freedom 2020; 4 Dec. https://www.scientificfreedom.dk/2020/12/04/the-coronavirus-has-created-a-nanny-state/.

[133] Ibid.

[134] Jefferson T. DR TOM JEFFERSON: As people test positive WEEKS after they stop being infectious, why I fear this mania for mass Covid testing is a hugely expensive blunder. Daily Mail 2020; 12 Dec.

[135] Ibid.

[136] Jefferson T, Spencer EA, Brassey J, Heneghan C. Viral cultures for COVID-19 infectious potential assessment - a systematic review. Clin Infect Dis 2020; 3 Dec. https://doi.org/10.1093/cid/ciaa1764.

[137] Shields A, Faustini SE, Perez-Toledo M, Jossi S, Aldera E, Allen JD, et al. SARS-CoV-2 seroprevalence and asymptomatic viral carriage in healthcare workers: a cross-sectional study. Thorax 2020;75:1089-94.

[138] Jefferson T. DR TOM JEFFERSON: As people test positive WEEKS after they stop being infectious, why I fear this mania for mass Covid testing is a hugely expensive blunder. Daily Mail 2020; 12 Dec.

[139] Gøtzsche PC. Deadly medicines and organised crime: How big pharma has corrupted health care. London: Radcliffe Publishing; 2013.; Gøtzsche PC. Deadly psychiatry and organised denial. Copenhagen: People's Press; 2015.

[140] Kendrick M. A health economic perspective on COVID-19. 2020; Mar 29. https://drmalcolmkendrick.org/2020/03/29/a-health-economic-perspective-on-covid-19/.

[141] Ibid.

[142] Aagaard LH. Sundhedsprofessor bryder tabu: Vi bruger "grotesk" mange penge på coronaen. Berlingske 2020; 5 Oct.

[143] Krumholz HM. Where have all the heart attacks gone? New York Times 2020; 6 Apr.

[144] CDC. Leading causes of death. https://www.cdc.gov/nchs/fastats/leading-causes-of-death.htm.

[145] Roberton T, Carter ED, Chou VB, Stegmuller AR, Jackson BD, Tam Y, et al. Early estimates of the indirect effects of the COVID-19 pandemic on maternal and child mortality in low-income and middle-income countries: a modelling study. Lancet Glob Health 2020;8:e901-8.

[146] COVID-19 to add as many as 150 million extreme poor by 2021. World Bank 2010; 7 Oct. https://www.worldbank.org/en/news/press-release/2020/10/07/covid-19-to-add-as-many-as-150-million-extreme-poor-by-2021.

[147] Kuloo M. "Hunger will kill us before coronavirus does": Migrant labourers in Kashmir say incomes have dried up and relief shelters are inadequate. Firstpost 2020; 8 Apr.

[148] Kendrick M. A health economic perspective on COVID-19. 2020; Mar 29. https://drmalcolmkendrick.org/2020/03/29/a-health-economic-perspective-on-covid-19/.

[149] Knapton S. Lockdown may cost 200,000 lives, government report shows. The Telegraph 2020; 19 July.

[150] Simon NM, Saxe GN, Marmar CR. Mental health disorders related to COVID-19–related deaths. JAMA 2020;324:1493-4.

[151] Ibid.

[152] Gøtzsche PC. Deadly psychiatry and organised denial. Copenhagen: People's Press; 2015.

[153] Hengartner MP, Plöderl M. Reply to the Letter to the Editor: "Newer-Generation Antidepressants and Suicide Risk: Thoughts on Hengartner and Plöderl's ReAnalysis." Psychother Psychosom 2019;88:373-4.; Gøtzsche PC. Mental health survival kit and withdrawal from psychiatric drugs. Copenhagen: Institute for Scientific Freedom; 2020.

[154] Gøtzsche PC, Gøtzsche PK. Cognitive behavioural therapy halves the risk of repeated suicide attempts: systematic review. J R Soc Med 2017;110:404-10.

[155] US antidepressant fills increased 20%; HCQ rose 525%. The Pharma Letter 2020; 19 Dec.

[156] Lenzer J, Brownlee S. The COVID science wars. Shutting down scientific debate is hurting the public health. Scientific American 2020; 30 Nov.

[157] Great Barington Declaration. 2020; 4 Oct. https://gbdeclaration.org/#sign.

[158] Alwan NA, Burgess RA, Ashworth S, Beale R, Bhadelia N, Bogaert D, Dowd J, et al. Scientific consensus on the COVID-19 pandemic: we need to act now. Lancet 2020;396:e71-2.

[159] Clark A, Jit M, Warren-Gash C, Guthrie B, Wang HHX, Mercer SW, et al. Global, regional, and national estimates of the population at increased risk of severe COVID-19 due to underlying health conditions in 2020: a modelling study. Lancet Glob Health 2020;8:e1003-17.

[160] Lenzer J, Brownlee S. The COVID science wars. Shutting down scientific debate is hurting the public health. Scientific American 2020; 30 Nov.

[161] Ibid.; Lenzer J, Brownlee S. The Ioannidis affair: a tale of major scientific overreaction. Scientific American 2020; 30 Nov.

[162] Lenzer J, Brownlee S. The Ioannidis affair: a tale of major scientific overreaction. Scientific American 2020; 30 Nov.

[163] Jamison P. A top scientist questioned virus lockdowns on Fox News. The backlash was fierce. Washington Post 2020; 16 Dec.

[164] Lenzer J, Brownlee S. The COVID science wars. Shutting down scientific debate is hurting the public health. Scientific American 2020; 30 Nov.

[165] Lenzer J, Brownlee S. The Ioannidis affair: a tale of major scientific overreaction. Scientific American 2020; 30 Nov.

[166] Lenzer J, Brownlee S. The COVID science wars. Shutting down scientific debate is hurting the public health. Scientific American 2020; 30 Nov.

[167] Ioannidis JPA. Infection fatality rate of COVID-19. Bull World Health Organ 2021 (in press).

[168] Lenzer J. The Scientific American dustup. https://jeannelenzer.com/scientific-american-scandal.

[169] Lenzer J. The Scientific American dustup. https://jeannelenzer.com/scientific-american-scandal.

[170] Ibid.

171 Gøtzsche PC. Serious editorial misconduct at Scientific American related to COVID-19. Institute for Scientific Freedom 2021; Jan. 1. https://www.scientificfreedom.dk/?p=1384&preview=true.

172 Aagaard LH. Professor: Stort dansk maskestudie afvist af tre top-tidsskrifter. *Berlingske* 2020; Oct. 22.

173 Lenzer J, Brownlee S. The COVID science wars. Shutting down scientific debate is hurting the public health. *Scientific American* 2020; Nov. 30.

174 Sodha S. We need scientists to quiz Covid consensus, not act as agents of disinformation. *The Guardian* 2020; Nov. 22.

175 Ioannidis JPA. A fiasco in the making? As the coronavirus pandemic takes hold, we are making decisions without reliable data.

176 Lenzer J, Brownlee S. The COVID science wars. Shutting down scientific debate is hurting the public health.

177 Abbassi K. Covid-19: politicisation, "corruption," and suppression of science. *BMJ* 2020;371:m4425.

178 Oxford COVID-19 Evidence Service. Regularly updated. https://www.cebm.net/covid-19/.

179 Doshi P. Calibrated response to emerging infections. *BMJ* 2009;339:b3471.

180 Ibid.

181 Gigerenzer G. Why what does not kill us makes us panic. 2020; Mar. 12. https://www.project-syndicate.org/commentary/greater-risk-literacy-can-reduce-coronavirus-fear-by-gerd-gigerenzer-2020-03.

182 Interview with John Ioannidis. YouTube 2020; Mar. 26. https://www.youtube.com/watch?v=d6MZy-2fcBw&t=1858s.

183 Patrick DM, Petric M, Skowronski DM, Guasparini R, Booth TF, Krajden M, et al. An outbreak of human Coronavirus OC43 infection and serological cross-reactivity with SARS Coronavirus. *Can J Infect Dis Med Microbiol* 2006;17:330–6.

184 Bendavid E, Oh C, Bhattacharya J, Ioannidis JPA. Assessing mandatory stay-at-home and business closure effects on the spread of COVID-19. Eur J Clin Invest 2021;51:e13484.

185 Packer G. We are living in a failed state. *The Atlantic* 2020; June.

186 Gøtzsche PC. *Deadly medicines and organised crime: How big pharma has corrupted health care*. London: Radcliffe Publishing; 2013.

187 Wealth but not health in the USA. *Lancet* 2013;381:177.

188 Baden LR, El Sahly HM, Essink B, Kotloff K, Frey S, Novak S, et al. Efficacy and safety of the mRNA-1273 SARS-CoV-2 vaccine. *N Engl J Med* 2020; Dec. 30. DOI: 10.1056/NEJMe2035557.

189 Roehr B. Health care in US ranks lowest among developed countries, Commonwealth Fund study shows. *BMJ* 2008;337:a889.

190 Brownlee S. *Overtreated: why too much medicine is making us sicker and poorer*. New York: Bloomsbury; 2007.

191 Obama B. *A promised land*. New York: Crown; 2020.

192 Friedman TL. Joe Biden, not Bernie Sanders, is the true Scandinavian. *New York Times* 2020; Mar. 10.

193 Kessler G, Rizzo S, Kelly M. President Trump has made more than 20,000 false or misleading claims. *Washington Post* 2020; July 13.

194 Obama B. *A promised land*.

195 Barrett T, Raju M, Nickeas P. US Capitol secured, 4 dead after rioters stormed the halls of Congress to block Biden's win. CNN 2020; Jan. 7.

CHAPTER 6

1   Gøtzsche PC. *Survival in an overmedicated world: look up the evidence yourself.* Copenhagen: People's Press; 2019.

2   Rasmussen LI. Hun kritiserede HPV-vaccinen og fik hug - nu giver hun op. *Politiken* 2016; Mar. 25.

3   European Medicines Agency. Assessment report. Review under Article 20 of Regulation (EC) No 726/2004. Human papilloma virus (HPV) vaccines. 2015; Nov. 11. http://www.ema.europa.eu/docs/en_GB/document_library/Referrals_document/HPV_vaccines_20/Opinion_provided_by_Committee_for_Medicinal_Products_for_Human_Use/WC500197129.pdf.

4   Brinth L, Theibel AC, Pors K, et al. Suspected side effects to the quadrivalent human papilloma vaccine. *Dan Med J* 2015;62:A5064; Brinth LS, Pors K, Theibel AC, et al. Orthostatic intolerance and postural tachycardia syndrome as suspected adverse effects of vaccination against human papilloma virus. *Vaccine* 2015;33:2602–5; Brinth L, Pors K, Hoppe AAG, et al. Is chronic fatigue syndrome/myalgic encephalomyelitis a relevant diagnosis in patients with suspected side effects to human papilloma virus vaccine? *Int J Vaccines Vaccin* 2015;1:00003.

5   Brinth L, Theibel AC, Pors K, et al. Suspected side effects to the quadrivalent human papilloma vaccine.

6   Ibid.

7   Fedorowski A, Li H, Yu X, et al. Antiadrenergic autoimmunity in postural tachycardia syndrome. *Europace* 2016; Oct 4. doi:10.1093/europace/euw154.

8   Mehlsen J, et al. Study of autoantibodies in HPV vaccinated patients. Presented at the 11th International Congress on Autoimmunity, Lisbon, Portugal. 2019; May 16–20. To be published.

9   Chandler RE. Modernising vaccine surveillance systems to improve detection of rare or poorly defined adverse events. *BMJ* 2019;365:l2268.

10 Brinth L, Theibel AC, Pors K, et al. Suspected side effects to the quadrivalent human papilloma vaccine.

11 Brinth LS, Pors K, Theibel AC, et al. Orthostatic intolerance and postural tachycardia syndrome as suspected adverse effects of vaccination against human papilloma virus.

12 Brinth L, Pors K, Hoppe AAG, et al. Is chronic fatigue syndrome/myalgic encephalomyelitis a relevant diagnosis in patients with suspected side effects to human papilloma virus vaccine?

13 European Medicines Agency. Assessment report. Review under Article 20 of Regulation (EC) No 726/2004. Human papilloma virus (HPV) vaccines.

14 Trojaborg K. Danske forskere sables ned: Ingen sammenhæng mellem HPV vaccine og alvorlige symptomer. Det Europæiske Lægemiddelagentur retter skarp kritik mod danske forskeres metoder. *Politiken* 2015; Nov. 26.

15 Rasmussen LI. Hun kritiserede HPV-vaccinen og fik hug - nu giver hun op.

16 European Medicines Agency. Assessment report. Review under Article 20 of Regulation (EC) No 726/2004. Human papilloma virus (HPV) vaccines.

17 Brinth L, Theibel AC, Pors K, et al. Suspected side effects to the quadrivalent human papilloma vaccine.

18 Rasmussen LI. Hun kritiserede HPV-vaccinen og fik hug - nu giver hun op.

19 Corfixen K. Liselott Blixt affejer HPV-rapport: "Lavet af betalt lobby." På trods af EMA-kritik stoler DF's udvalgsformand stadig fuldt ud på dansk HPV-center. *Politiken* 2015; Nov. 26.

20 Funch SM. "Journalistik som det her risikerer i sidste ende at koste liv." *Journalisten* 2016; June 11.

21 European Medicines Agency. Assessment report. Review under Article 20 of Regulation (EC) No 726/2004. Human papilloma virus (HPV) vaccines.

22 Gøtzsche PC, Jørgensen KJ, Jefferson T, et al. Complaint to the European Medicines Agency (EMA) over maladministration at the EMA. 2016; May 25. http://www .deadlymedicines.dk/wp-content/uploads/2019/02/10.-2016-05-26-Complaint-to -EMA-over-EMAs-handling-of-safety-of-the-HPV-vaccines.pdf.

23 Briefing note to experts. EMA/666938/2015. 2015; Oct. 13. http://ijme.in/pdf/g -briefing-note-to-the-experts-ema-oct-2015-unredacted.pdf.

24 European Medicines Agency. Assessment report. Review under Article 20 of Regulation (EC) No 726/2004. Human papilloma virus (HPV) vaccines; Gøtzsche PC, Jørgensen KJ, Jefferson T, et al. Complaint to the European Medicines Agency (EMA) over maladministration at the EMA; Briefing note to experts; Gøtzsche PC, Jørgensen KJ, Jefferson T, et al. Complaint to the European ombudsman over maladministration at the European Medicines Agency (EMA) in relation to the safety of the HPV vaccines. 2016; Oct. 10. http://www.deadlymedicines.dk/wp-content/uploads/2019/02/8.-2016-10-10 -Complaint-to-the-EU-ombudsman-over-the-EMA.pdf.

25 Gøtzsche PC, Jørgensen KJ. Mishandling the suspected serious neurological harms from the HPV vaccines by EMA. *BMJ Evid Based Med* 2021 (in press). See also: https://www .deadlymedicines.dk/complaint-to-the-european-ombudsman/.

26 Gøtzsche PC. *Deadly medicines and organised crime: How big pharma has corrupted health care.* London: Radcliffe Publishing; 2013; Gøtzsche PC. *Deadly psychiatry and organised denial.* Copenhagen: People's Press; 2015.

27 Briefing note to experts. EMA/666938/2015.

28 European Medicines Agency. Assessment report. Review under Article 20 of Regulation (EC) No 726/2004. Human papilloma virus (HPV) vaccines.

29 Briefing note to experts. EMA/666938/2015.

30 Gøtzsche PC, Jørgensen KJ, Jefferson T, et al. Complaint to the European ombudsman over maladministration at the European Medicines Agency (EMA) in relation to the safety of the HPV vaccines.

31 Ibid; Jefferson T, Jørgensen L. Human papillomavirus vaccines, complex regional pain syndrome, postural orthostatic tachycardia syndrome, and autonomic dysfunction – a review of the regulatory evidence from the European Medicines Agency.

32 Weber C, Andersen S. Firma bag HPV-vaccinen underdrev omfanget af alvorlige bivirkninger. *Berlingske* 2015; Oct. 26.

33 Dunder K, Mueller-Berghaus J. Rapporteurs' Day 150 Joint Response Assessment Report. *Gardasil 9.* 2014; Nov. 23.

34 Joelving F. What the Gardasil testing may have missed. *Slate* 2017; Dec. 17.

35 Dunder K, Mueller-Berghaus J. Rapporteurs' Day 150 Joint Response Assessment Report.

36 Joelving F. What the Gardasil testing may have missed.

37 Ibid.

38 Ibid.

39 Ibid.

40 Ibid.

41 Dunder K, Mueller-Berghaus J. Rapporteurs' Day 150 Joint Response Assessment Report.

42 Joelving F. What the Gardasil testing may have missed.

43 FUTURE II Study Group. Quadrivalent vaccine against human papillomavirus to prevent high-grade cervical lesions. *N Engl J Med* 2007;356:1915–27.

44 Gøtzsche PC, Jørgensen KJ, Jefferson T, et al. Complaint to the European ombudsman over maladministration at the European Medicines Agency (EMA) in relation to the safety of the HPV vaccines.

45 Gøtzsche PC, Jørgensen KJ, Jefferson T, et al. Our comment on the decision by the European Ombudsman about our complaint over maladministration at the European Medicines Agency related to safety of the HPV vaccines. 2017; Nov. 2. http://www .deadlymedicines.dk/wp-content/uploads/2019/02/1.-2017-11-02-Our-assessment-on -the-Ombudsmans-decision.pdf.

46 European Medicines Agency. Assessment report. Review under Article 20 of Regulation (EC) No 726/2004. Human papilloma virus (HPV) vaccines.

47 Briefing note to experts. EMA/666938/2015.

48 Ibid.

49 Gøtzsche PC, Jørgensen KJ, Jefferson T, et al. Complaint to the European Medicines Agency (EMA) over maladministration at the EMA.

50 Jørgensen L, Gøtzsche PC, Jefferson T. Benefits and harms of the human papillomavirus (HPV) vaccines: systematic review with meta-analyses of trial data from clinical study reports. Syst Rev 2020;9:43. The data can also be found here: Jørgensen L. Benefits and Harms of the Human Papillomavirus (HPV) Vaccines. PhD thesis defended Mar. 12, 2019, at the University of Copenhagen. http://bit.ly/PhDHPVvaccines.

51 A study of V503, a 9-valent human papillomavirus (9vHPV) vaccine in females 12–26 years of age who have previously received GARDASIL™ (V503-006). https: //clinicaltrials.gov/show/NCT01047345.

52 Briefing note to experts. EMA/666938/2015; Gøtzsche PC, Jørgensen KJ, Jefferson T, et al. Complaint to the European ombudsman over maladministration at the European Medicines Agency (EMA) in relation to the safety of the HPV vaccines.

53 European Medicines Agency. Assessment report. Review under Article 20 of Regulation (EC) No 726/2004. Human papilloma virus (HPV) vaccines.

54 Briefing note to experts. EMA/666938/2015.

55 Jørgensen L, Gøtzsche PC, Jefferson T. The Cochrane HPV vaccine review was incomplete and ignored important evidence of bias: Response to the Cochrane editors. 2018; Sept. 17. https://ebm.bmj.com/content/early/2018/07/27/bmjebm-2018-111012.responses# the-cochrane-hpvvaccine-review-was-incomplete-and-ignored-important-evidence -of-bias-response-to-the-cochraneeditors; Expert consultation on the use of placebos in vaccine trials. WHO 2013. https://apps.who.int/iris/bitstream/handle/10665/94056 /9789241506250_eng.pdf?sequence=1.

56 Thiriot DS, Ahl PL, Cannon J, et al. Method for preparation of aluminium hydroxyphosphate adjuvant. Patent WO2013078102A1. 2013; 30 May. https://patents .google.com/patent/WO2013078102A1/en.

57 Jørgensen L, Gøtzsche PC, Jefferson T. The Cochrane HPV vaccine review was incomplete and ignored important evidence of bias: Response to the Cochrane editors.

58 FDA approved package insert for Gardasil, first approved in 2006. https://www.fda.gov /files/vaccines,%20blood%20&%20biologics/published/Package-Insert-Gardasil.pdf.

59 Gøtzsche PC, Jørgensen KJ, Jefferson T, et al. Our comment on the decision by the European Ombudsman about our complaint over maladministration at the European Medicines Agency related to safety of the HPV vaccines.

60 Ibid.

61 http://www.who.int/vaccine_safety/committee/reports/Jun_2012/en/index.html.

62 Beppu H, Minaguchi M, Uchide K, et al. Lessons learnt in Japan from adverse reactions to the HPV vaccine: a medical ethics perspective. *Indian J Med Ethics* 2017;2:82–8.

63 Masson JD, Crépeaux G, Authier FJ, et al. Critical analysis of reference studies on the toxicokinetics of aluminium-based adjuvants. *J Inorg Biochem* 2018;181:87–95.

64 Jørgensen L, Gøtzsche PC, Jefferson T. The Cochrane HPV vaccine review was incomplete and ignored important evidence of bias: Response to the Cochrane editors; Thiriot DS, Ahl PL, Cannon J, et al. Method for preparation of aluminium hydroxyphosphate adjuvant.

65 Liang XF, Wang HQ, Wang JZ, et al. Safety and immunogenicity of 2009 pandemic influenza A H1N1 vaccines in China: a multicentre, double–blind, randomised, placebo-controlled trial. *Lancet* 2010;375:56–66.

66 Masson JD, Crépeaux G, Authier FJ, et al. Critical analysis of reference studies on the toxicokinetics of aluminium-based adjuvants.

67 Asín J, Pérez M, Pinczowski P. From the bluetongue vaccination campaigns in sheep to overimmunization and ovine ASIA syndrome. *Immunologic Res* 2019. https://doi .org/10.1007/s12026-018-9059-7.

68 Luján L, Pérez M, Salazar E, et al. Autoimmune/autoinflammatory syndrome induced by adjuvants (ASIA syndrome) in commercial sheep. *Immunol Res* 2013;56:317–24.

69 Asín J, Pérez M, Pinczowski P. From the bluetongue vaccination campaigns in sheep to overimmunization and ovine ASIA syndrome.

70 Asín J, Pascual-Alonsob M, Pinczowski P, et al. Cognition and behavior in sheep repetitively inoculated with aluminium adjuvant-containing vaccines or aluminium adjuvant only. *Pharmacol Res* 2018; Nov. 3. pii: S1043-6618(18)31373-2. doi: 10.1016/j.phrs.2018.10.019. (Epub ahead of print.) Retracted by Elsevier without any explanation, see: https://www.sciencedirect.com/science/article/pii/S104 3661818313732?via%3Dihub.

71 Ibid.

72 Hawkes D, Benhamu J, Sidwell T, et al. Revisiting adverse reactions to vaccines: A critical appraisal of Autoimmune Syndrome Induced by Adjuvants (ASIA). *J Autoimmun* 2015;59:77–84.

73 Asín J, Pascual-Alonsob M, Pinczowski P, et al. Cognition and behavior in sheep repetitively inoculated with aluminium adjuvant-containing vaccines or aluminium adjuvant only.

74 Wager E, Barbour V, Yentis S, et al. Retractions: Guidance from the Committee on Publication Ethics (COPE). *Croat Med J* 2009;50:532–5.

75 International Committee of Medical Journal Editors. Scientific misconduct, expressions of concern, and retraction. http://www.icmje.org/recommendations/browse/publishing -and-editorial-issues/scientific-misconduct-expressions-of-concern-and-retraction.html.

76 Kell G. Why UC split with publishing giant Elsevier. 2019; Mar. 6. https://www .universityofcalifornia.edu/news/why-uc-split-publishing-giant-elsevier.

77 Gonzalez R. The wealthiest university on Earth can't afford its academic journal subscriptions. *Gizmodo* 2012; Apr. 24.

78 Briefing note to experts. EMA/666938/2015.

79 PRAC (co-)rapporteur's referral 2nd Updated preliminary assessment report. 2015; Oct. 28. https://www.deadlymedicines.dk/wp-content/uploads/29-Co-Rapporteur-2nd -Updated-assessment-report.pdf.

80   Gøtzsche PC, Jørgensen KJ, Jefferson T, et al. Our comment on the decision by the European Ombudsman about our complaint over maladministration at the European Medicines Agency related to safety of the HPV vaccines.

81   Ibid.

82   Benarroch EE. Postural tachycardia syndrome: a heterogeneous and multifactorial disorder. *Mayo Clin Proc* 2012;87:1214–25.

83   Ibid.

84   Gøtzsche PC, Jørgensen KJ, Jefferson T, et al. Our comment on the decision by the European Ombudsman about our complaint over maladministration at the European Medicines Agency related to safety of the HPV vaccines; European Ombudsman. Decision in case 1475/2016/JAS on the European Medicines Agency's handling of the referral procedure relating to human papillomavirus (HPV) vaccines. 2017; Oct. 16. https://www.ombudsman.europa.eu/cases/decision.faces/en/84736/html.bookmark.

85   Dirckx M, Schreurs MW, de Mos M, et al. The prevalence of autoantibodies in complex regional pain syndrome type I. *Mediators Inflamm* 2015;2015:718201.

86   European Ombudsman. Decision in case 1475/2016/JAS on the European Medicines Agency's handling of the referral procedure relating to human papillomavirus (HPV) vaccines.

87   European Medicines Agency. Assessment report. Review under Article 20 of Regulation (EC) No 726/2004. Human papilloma virus (HPV) vaccines.

88   Briefing note to experts. EMA/666938/2015; Gøtzsche PC, Jørgensen KJ, Jefferson T, et al. Our comment on the decision by the European Ombudsman about our complaint over maladministration at the European Medicines Agency related to safety of the HPV vaccines.

89   European Medicines Agency. Assessment report. Review under Article 20 of Regulation (EC) No 726/2004. Human papilloma virus (HPV) vaccines.

90   Letter from the European Ombudsman to the Nordic Cochrane Centre. 2017; June 26. http://www.deadlymedicines.dk/wp-content/uploads/2019/02/4.-2017-06-26-Letter -from-Ombudsman-to-Nordic-Cochrane-Centre.pdf.

91   Gøtzsche PC, Jørgensen KJ, Jefferson T, et al. Our comment on the decision by the European Ombudsman about our complaint over maladministration at the European Medicines Agency related to safety of the HPV vaccines.

92   Briefing note to experts. EMA/666938/2015.

93   European Medicines Agency. Assessment report. Review under Article 20 of Regulation (EC) No 726/2004. Human papilloma virus (HPV) vaccines.

94   Gøtzsche PC, Jørgensen KJ, Jefferson T, et al. Our comment on the decision by the European Ombudsman about our complaint over maladministration at the European Medicines Agency related to safety of the HPV vaccines.

95   Butts BN, Fischer PR, Mack KJ. Human papillomavirus vaccine and postural orthostatic tachycardia syndrome: a review of current literature. *J Child Neurol* 2017;32:956–65.

96   European Medicines Agency. Assessment report. Review under Article 20 of Regulation (EC) No 726/2004. Human papilloma virus (HPV) vaccines.

97   Ibid.

98   Briefing note to experts. EMA/666938/2015.

99   PRAC (co-)rapporteur's referral 2nd Updated preliminary assessment report.

100   European Medicines Agency. Assessment report. Review under Article 20 of Regulation (EC) No 726/2004. Human papilloma virus (HPV) vaccines.

101   Briefing note to experts. EMA/666938/2015.

[102] European Medicines Agency. Assessment report. Review under Article 20 of Regulation (EC) No 726/2004. Human papilloma virus (HPV) vaccines.

[103] Briefing note to experts. EMA/666938/2015.

[104] Ibid; European Medicines Agency. Assessment report. Review under Article 20 of Regulation (EC) No 726/2004. Human papilloma virus (HPV) vaccines.

[105] Gøtzsche PC, Jørgensen KJ, Jefferson T, et al. Complaint to the European ombudsman over maladministration at the European Medicines Agency (EMA) in relation to the safety of the HPV vaccines.

[106] Chandler RE, Juhlin K, Fransson J, et al. Current safety concerns with human papillomavirus vaccine: a cluster analysis of reports in Vigibase (R). *Drug Saf* 2017;40:81–90.

[107] Letter from EMA to the Nordic Cochrane Centre. 2016; 1 July. http://www.ema.europa.eu/docs/en_GB/document_library/Other/2016/07/WC500210543.pdf.

[108] Gøtzsche PC, Jørgensen KJ, Jefferson T, et al. Complaint to the European ombudsman over maladministration at the European Medicines Agency (EMA) in relation to the safety of the HPV vaccines.

[109] Ibid; Letter from EMA to the Nordic Cochrane Centre.

[110] European Ombudsman. Decision in case 1475/2016/JAS on the European Medicines Agency's handling of the referral procedure relating to human papillomavirus (HPV) vaccines.

[111] Gøtzsche PC, Jørgensen KJ, Jefferson T, et al. Complaint to the European ombudsman over maladministration at the European Medicines Agency (EMA) in relation to the safety of the HPV vaccines.

[112] Gøtzsche PC. *Deadly medicines and organised crime: How big pharma has corrupted health care.*

[113] Ibid.

[114] European Ombudsman. *Decision in case 1606/2016/JAS* on the European Medicines Agency's handling of an alleged failure to declare interests by its Executive Director. 2017; Nov. 22. https://www.ombudsman.europa.eu/en/decision/en/86541.

[115] Head MG, Wind-Mozley M, Flegg PJ. Inadvisable anti-vaccination sentiment: Human Papilloma Virus immunisation falsely under the microscope. *NPJ Vaccines* 2017 Mar. 8;2:6. doi: 10.1038/s41541-017-0004-x. eCollection 2017.

[116] https://twitter.com/lmstsenderovitz?lang=en.

[117] https://twitter.com/OleToftSundhed/status/841914715509010433.

[118] https://twitter.com/search?q=%22How%20easy%20is%20misinformation%3F%.3F%3F%E2%80%9D&src=typed_query.

[119] https://twitter.com/search?q=%22Og%20de%20kritiserer%20altid%20andre%20-for%20inhabilitet!%22&src=typed_query&f=live.

[120] https://twitter.com/search?q=%22Nature%20om%20HPV%22&src=typed_query.

[121] https://twitter.com/OleToftSundhed/status/841914715509010433.

[122] https://www.facebook.com/poul.videbech.

[123] https://www.facebook.com/519677024898789/posts/605754569624367/.

[124] https://twitter.com/OleToftSundhed/status/841914715509010433.

[125] Arbyn M, Xu L, Simoens C, et al. Prophylactic vaccination against human papillomaviruses to prevent cervical cancer and its precursors. *Cochrane Database Syst Rev* 2018;5:CD009069.

126 Arbyn M, Bryant A, Beutels P, et al. Prophylactic vaccination against human papilloma-viruses to prevent cervical cancer and its precursors (protocol). *Cochrane Database Syst Rev* 2011;4:CD009069.

127 Cochrane Collaboration policy on commercial sponsorship of Cochrane reviews and Cochrane groups. 2014; Mar. 8. http://community.cochrane.org/organisational-policy-manual/appendix-5-commercial-sponsorship-policy.

128 Ibid.

129 Ibid.

130 Gøtzsche PC. Cochrane authors on drug industry payroll should not be allowed. *BMJ Evid Based Med* 2019; Apr. 11. pii: bmjebm-2018-111124. doi: 10.1136/bmjebm-2018-111124. (Epub ahead of print.)

131 Jørgensen L, Gøtzsche PC, Jefferson T. The Cochrane HPV vaccine review was incomplete and ignored important evidence of bias. *BMJ Evid Based Med* 2018;23:165–8.

132 Arbyn M, Bryant A, Beutels P, et al. Prophylactic vaccination against human papillomaviruses to prevent cervical cancer and its precursors (protocol).

133 Jørgensen L, Gøtzsche PC, Jefferson T. The Cochrane HPV vaccine review was incomplete and ignored important evidence of bias: Response to the Cochrane editors.

134 Hawkes N. Cochrane examines whether lead author of HPV review had undeclared conflicts of interest. *BMJ* 2018;363;k4163.

135 Hawkes N. Lead author of Cochrane HPV review did not breach conflicts policy, find arbiters. *BMJ* 2018;363:k4352.

136 Ibid.

137 Jørgensen L, Gøtzsche PC, Jefferson T. The Cochrane HPV vaccine review was incomplete and ignored important evidence of bias.

138 Krause P. Update on vaccine regulation: expediting vaccine development. 2014; May 5. https://cdn.ymaws.com/www.casss.org/resource/resmgr/CMC_Euro_Speaker_Slides/2014_CMCE_KrausePhil.pdf.

139 Jørgensen L, Gøtzsche PC, Jefferson T. The Cochrane HPV vaccine review was incomplete and ignored important evidence of bias.

140 Ibid.

141 Chandler RE, Juhlin K, Fransson J, et al. Current safety concerns with human papillomavirus vaccine: a cluster analysis of reports in Vigibase (R).

142 Jørgensen L, Gøtzsche PC, Jefferson T. The Cochrane HPV vaccine review was incomplete and ignored important evidence of bias: Response to the Cochrane editors.

143 Demasi M. Cochrane – A sinking ship? 2018; Sept. 16. https://blogs.bmj.com/bmjebmspotlight/2018/09/16/cochrane-a-sinking-ship/.

144 Jørgensen L, Gøtzsche PC, Jefferson T. The Cochrane HPV vaccine review was incomplete and ignored important evidence of bias.

145 Gøtzsche PC. *Death of a whistleblower and Cochrane's moral collapse.* Copenhagen: People's Press; 2019.

146 Tovey D, Soares-Weiser K. Cochrane's Editor in Chief responds to BMJ EBM article criticizing HPV review. 2018; Sept. 3. https://www.cochrane.org/news/cochranes-editor-chief-responds-bmj-ebm-article-criticizing-hpv-review.

147 Schopenhauer A. *The art of always being right.* London: Gibson Square; 2009.

148 Jørgensen L, Gøtzsche PC, Jefferson T. The Cochrane HPV vaccine review was incomplete and ignored important evidence of bias: Response to the Cochrane editors.

149 Ibid.

150 Ibid.

[151] Tovey D, Soares-Weiser K. Cochrane's Editor in Chief responds to BMJ EBM article criticizing HPV review.

[152] Gøtzsche PC. *Death of a whistleblower and Cochrane's moral collapse.*

[153] Ibid.

[154] Ibid.

[155] Jørgensen L, Gøtzsche PC, Jefferson T. Benefits and harms of the human papillomavirus (HPV) vaccines: systematic review with meta-analyses of trial data from clinical study reports.

[156] Ibid.

[157] Ibid.

[158] Ibid.

[159] Jefferson T, Jørgensen L. Human papillomavirus vaccines, complex regional pain syndrome, postural orthostatic tachycardia syndrome, and autonomic dysfunction – a review of the regulatory evidence from the European Medicines Agency.

[160] Jørgensen L, Gøtzsche PC, Jefferson T. Index of the human papillomavirus (HPV) vaccine industry clinical study programmes and non-industry funded studies: a necessary basis to address reporting bias in a systematic review. *Syst Rev* 2018;7:8.

[161] Jørgensen L, Gøtzsche PC, Jefferson T. Benefits and harms of the human papillomavirus (HPV) vaccines: systematic review with meta-analyses of trial data from clinical study reports.

[162] Ibid.

[163] Dalgas J. KU godkender kontroversiel HPV-forskning: "Handler det om, at man vil promovere en eller anden anti-vaccinedagsorden?" *Berlingske* 2019; Mar. 15.

[164] TV2. De vaccinerede piger. 2015; Mar. 26.

[165] Højsgaard L. Myndigheder: Mediernes stærke HPV-cases kan overdøve fakta. *Journalisten* 2017; May 10.

[166] Chandler RE, Juhlin K, Fransson J, et al. Current safety concerns with human papillomavirus vaccine: a cluster analysis of reports in Vigibase (R).

[167] https://www.information.dk/debat/2017/02/fake-news-lodret-skraemmepropaganda -propaganda-tages-ved-roden

[168] Johnsen PP. Håret i den medicinske suppe. *Weekendavisen* 2018; Feb. 2.

[169] Gøtzsche PC, Jørgensen KJ, Jefferson T, et al. Our comment on the decision by the European Ombudsman about our complaint over maladministration at the European Medicines Agency related to safety of the HPV vaccines.

[170] Kyrgiou M, Athanasiou A, Paraskevaidi M, et al. Adverse obstetric outcomes after local treatment for cervical preinvasive and early invasive disease according to cone depth: systematic review and meta-analysis. *BMJ* 2016;354:i3633.

[171] Arbyn M, Xu L, Simoens C, et al. Prophylactic vaccination against human papillomaviruses to prevent cervical cancer and its precursors.

[172] Cervical cancer: abnormal cells on the cervix (dysplasia). 2017; Dec. 14. https://www .ncbi.nlm.nih.gov/books/NBK279256/.

[173] Palmer T, Wallace L, Pollock KG, et al. Prevalence of cervical disease at age 20 after immunisation with bivalent HPV vaccine at age 12–13 in Scotland: retrospective population study. *BMJ* 2019;365:l1161.

[174] Drolet M, Bénard É, Pérez N, et al. Population-level impact and herd effects following the introduction of human papillomavirus vaccination programmes: updated systematic review and meta-analysis. *Lancet* 2019;394:497–509.

[175] Martínez-Lavín M, Amezcua-Guerra L. Serious adverse events after HPV vaccination: a critical review of randomized trials and post-marketing case series. *Clin Rheumatol* 2017;36:2169–78.

[176] Joura EA, Giuliano AR, Iversen OE, et al. A 9-valent HPV vaccine against infection and intraepithelial neoplasia in women. *N Engl J Med* 2015;372:711–23.

[177] Ibid; Martínez-Lavín M, Amezcua-Guerra L. Serious adverse events after HPV vaccination: a critical review of randomized trials and post-marketing case series.

[178] Joura EA, Giuliano AR, Iversen OE, et al. A 9-valent HPV vaccine against infection and intraepithelial neoplasia in women.

[179] Ibid.

[180] Ibid.

[181] Jørgensen L, Gøtzsche PC, Jefferson T. The Cochrane HPV vaccine review was incomplete and ignored important evidence of bias: Response to the Cochrane editors.

[182] Capilla A. Justice recognizes what health authorities do not want to recognize. 2017; Apr. 16. http://sanevax.org/hpv-vaccine-death-spain/.

[183] From a letter sent by a researcher from my HPV research group to the Uppsala Monitoring Centre on July 7, 2017.

[184] Tozzi AE, Asturias EJ, Balakrishnan MR, et al. Assessment of causality of individual adverse events following immunization (AEFI): a WHO tool for global use. *Vaccine* 2013;31:5041–6.

[185] Puliyel J, Phadke A. Deaths following pentavalent vaccine and the revised AEFI classification. *Indian J Med Ethics* 2017; July 4.

[186] Ibid; Tozzi AE, Asturias EJ, Balakrishnan MR, et al. Assessment of causality of individual adverse events following immunization (AEFI): a WHO tool for global use.

[187] Donegan K, Beau-Lejdstrom R, King B, et al. Bivalent human papillomavirus vaccine and the risk of fatigue syndromes in girls in the UK. *Vaccine* 2013;31:4961–7.

[188] Gallagher P. Thousands of teenage girls report feeling seriously ill after routine school cancer vaccination. *The Independent* 2015; May 31.

[189] Joura EA, Giuliano AR, Iversen OE, et al. A 9-valent HPV vaccine against infection and intraepithelial neoplasia in women.

[190] Hoffmann T. Kritik hagler ned over nyt HPV-studie. 2017; Sept. 12. Videnskab.dk.

[191] Scheller NM, Svanström H, Pasternak B, et al. Quadrivalent HPV vaccination and risk of multiple sclerosis and other demyelinating diseases of the central nervous system. *JAMA* 2015;313:54–61.

[192] Mølbak K, Hansen ND, Valentiner-Branth P. Pre-vaccination care-seeking in females reporting severe adverse reactions to hpv vaccine. a registry based case-control study. *PLoS One* 2016;11:e0162520.

[193] Grönlund O, Herweijer E, Sundström K, et al. Incidence of new-onset autoimmune disease in girls and women with pre-existing autoimmune disease after quadrivalent human papillomavirus vaccination: a cohort study. *J Intern Med* 2016;280:618–26.

[194] Chandler RE. Modernising vaccine surveillance systems to improve detection of rare or poorly defined adverse events.

[195] Arana J, Mba-Jonas A, Jankosky C, et al. Reports of Postural Orthostatic Tachycardia Syndrome after human papillomavirus vaccination in the Vaccine Adverse Event Reporting System. *J Adolesc Health* 2017;61:577–82.

[196] Slade BA, Leidel L, Vellozzi C, et al. Postlicensure safety surveillance for quadrivalent human papillomavirus recombinant vaccine. *JAMA* 2009;302:750–7.

197 Kinoshita T, Abe RT, Hineno A, et al. Peripheral sympathetic nerve dysfunction in adolescent Japanese girls following immunization with the human papillomavirus vaccine. *Intern Med* 2014;53:2185–200.

198 Brinth LS, Pors K, Theibel AC, et al. Orthostatic intolerance and postural tachycardia syndrome as suspected adverse effects of vaccination against human papilloma virus.

199 Lareb. Long-lasting adverse events following immunization with Cervarix. 2015. http://databankws.lareb.nl/Downloads/Lareb_rapport_HPV_dec15_03.pdf.

200 European Medicines Agency. Assessment report. Review under Article 20 of Regulation (EC) No 726/2004. Human papilloma virus (HPV) vaccines.

201 CDC. HPV vaccine is cancer prevention for boys, too! https://www.cdc.gov/features/hpvvaccineboys/index.html.

202 Krogsbøll LT, Jørgensen KJ, Gøtzsche PC. General health checks in adults for reducing morbidity and mortality from disease. *Cochrane Database Syst Rev* 2019;1:CD009009.

203 CDC. Cancer deaths in the US. https://seer.cancer.gov/archive/csr/1975_2015/results_merged/sect_01_overview.pdf.

CHAPTER 7

1 Gøtzsche PC. *Survival in an overmedicated world: look up the evidence yourself.* Copenhagen: People's Press; 2019.

2 WHO. Japanese encephalitis. 2019; May 9. https://www.who.int/news-room/fact-sheets/detail/japanese-encephalitis.

3 Ibid.

4 Nothdurft HD, Jelinek T, Marschang A, et al. Adverse reactions to Japanese encephalitis vaccine in travellers. *J Infect* 1996;32:119–22.

5 CDC. Japanese encephalitis. Updated May 14, 2019. https://wwwnc.cdc.gov/travel/diseases/japanese-encephalitis.

CHAPTER 8

1 Statens Seruminstitut. Det danske børnevaccinationsprogram. 2019; Mar. 7. https://www.ssi.dk/vaccinationer/boernevaccination.

2 CDC. Recommended child and adolescent immunization schedule for ages 18 years or younger, United States, 2019. https://www.cdc.gov/vaccines/schedules/hcp/imz/child-adolescent.html.

3 NHS. The complete routine immunisation schedule from autumn 2018. https://assets.publishing.service.gov.uk/government/uploads/system/uploads/attachment_data/file/741543/Complete_immunisation_schedule_sept2018.pdf.

4 Gøtzsche PC. *Deadly medicines and organised crime: How big pharma has corrupted health care.* London: Radcliffe Publishing; 2013.

5 Ibid.

6 Ibid; Gøtzsche PC. *Survival in an overmedicated world: look up the evidence yourself.* Copenhagen: People's Press; 2019.

7 Hib vaccine. https://en.wikipedia.org/wiki/Hib_vaccine.

8 Higgins JPT, Soares-Weiser K, Reingold A. Systematic review of the non-specific effects of BCG, DTP and measles containing vaccines. 2014; Mar. 13. https://www.who.int

/immunization/sage/meetings/2014/april/3_NSE_Epidemiology_review_Report_to
_SAGE_14_Mar_FINAL.pdf.

9   Mogensen SW, Andersen A, Rodrigues A, et al. The introduction of diphtheria-tetanus-
    pertussis and oral polio vaccine among young infants in an urban African community:
    a natural experiment. *EBioMedicine* 2017;17:192–8; Aaby P, Mogensen SW, Rodrigues
    A, et al. Evidence of increase in mortality after the introduction of diphtheria-tetanus-
    pertussis vaccine to children aged 6-35 months in Guinea-Bissau: a time for reflection?
    Front Public Health 2018;19:79.

10 Aaby P, Mogensen SW, Rodrigues A, et al. Evidence of increase in mortality after the
    introduction of diphtheria-tetanus-pertussis vaccine to children aged 6-35 months in
    Guinea-Bissau: a time for reflection?

11 Kahneman D. *Thinking, fast and slow.* London: Penguin Books; 2012.

12 Aaby P, Mogensen SW, Rodrigues A, et al. Evidence of increase in mortality after the
    introduction of diphtheria-tetanus-pertussis vaccine to children aged 6-35 months in
    Guinea-Bissau: a time for reflection?

13 Meeting of the Strategic Advisory Group of Experts on immunization, April 2014 –
    conclusions and Recommendations. Wkly Epidemiol Rec 2014;89:221–36. https:
    //www.who.int/wer/2014/wer8921.pdf?ua=1.

14 Aaby P, Mogensen SW, Rodrigues A, et al. Evidence of increase in mortality after the
    introduction of diphtheria-tetanus-pertussis vaccine to children aged 6-35 months in
    Guinea-Bissau: a time for reflection?

15 Demicheli V, Rivetti A, Debalini MG, et al. Vaccines for measles, mumps and rubella in
    children. *Cochrane Database Syst Rev* 2012;(2):CD004407.

16 Ibid; Miller E, Goldacre M, Pugh S, et al. Risk of aseptic meningitis after measles,
    mumps, and rubella vaccine in UK children. *Lancet* 1993;341:979–82.

17 Miller E, Goldacre M, Pugh S, et al. Risk of aseptic meningitis after measles, mumps,
    and rubella vaccine in UK children.

18 WHO. Safety of mumps vaccine strains. 2007; Jan. 19. https://www.who.int/vaccine
    _safety/committee/topics/mumps/Dec_2006/en/.

19 Brown EG, Furesz J, Dimock K, et al. Nucleotide sequence analysis of Urabe mumps
    vaccine strain that caused meningitis in vaccine recipients. *Vaccine* 1991;9:840–2.

20 https://childhealthsafety.wordpress.com/about/.

21 ChildHealthSafety. Secret British MMR vaccine files forced open by legal action.
    2009; Jan. 13. https://childhealthsafety.wordpress.com/2009/01/13/secret-british-mmr
    -vaccine-files-forced-open-by-legal-action/.

22 Demicheli V, Rivetti A, Debalini MG, et al. Vaccines for measles, mumps and rubella in
    children.

23 CDC. Measles. Undated. https://www.cdc.gov/vaccines/pubs/pinkbook/meas.html.

24 WHO. Poliomyelitis. https://www.who.int/news-room/fact-sheets/detail/poliomyelitis.

25 Beaubien J. Mutant strains of polio vaccine now cause more paralysis than
    wild polio. National Public Radio 2017; June 28. https://www.npr.org/sections
    /goatsandsoda/2017/06/28/534403083/mutant-strains-of-polio-vaccine-now-cause
    -more-paralysis-than-wild-polio.

26 Lund N, Andersen A, Hansen AS, et al. The effect of oral polio vaccine at birth on infant
    mortality: a randomized trial. *Clin Infect Dis* 2015;61:1504–11; Andersen A, Fisker AB,
    Rodrigues A, et al. National immunization campaigns with oral polio vaccine reduce
    all-cause mortality: a natural experiment within seven randomized trials. *Front Public
    Health* 2018;6:13.

27 WHO. Introduction of rotavirus vaccines. 2013; July 31. http://www.who.int
    /immunization/monitoring_surveillance/burden/vpd/surveillance_type/sentinel
    /rotavirus_intro_guidance_who_july31_2013.pdf.

28 Schwartz JL. The first rotavirus vaccine and the politics of acceptable risk. *Milbank Q*
    2012;90:278–310.

29 Ibid.

30 Ibid.

31 WHO. Introduction of rotavirus vaccines.

32 Schwartz JL. The first rotavirus vaccine and the politics of acceptable risk.

33 Ibid.

34 Gøtzsche PC. *Deadly medicines and organised crime: How big pharma has corrupted health
    care.*

35 WHO. Pneumococcal conjugate vaccines. Undated. https://www.who.int/biologicals
    /areas/vaccines/pneumo/en/.

36 Lucero MG, Dulalia VE, Nillos LT, et al. Pneumococcal conjugate vaccines for preventing
    vaccine-type invasive pneumococcal disease and X-ray defined pneumonia in children
    less than two years of age. *Cochrane Database Syst Rev* 2009;4:CD004977.

37 Moberley S, Holden J, Tatham DP, et al. Vaccines for preventing pneumococcal infection
    in adults. *Cochrane Database Syst Rev* 2013;1:CD000422.

38 CDC. Adults: Protect yourself with pneumococcal vaccines. 2018; Sept. 17. https:
    //www.cdc.gov/features/adult-pneumococcal/index.html.

39 Herman B. CDC walks back pneumonia vaccine recommendation for seniors. 2019;
    June 26. https://www.axios.com/cdc-vote-pneumococcal-vaccine-seniors-prevnar-pfizer
    -a3e56ec6-f0fd-45a1-a313-a459e51e7b00.html.

40 Stepko B. Recommendation for pneumonia vaccine revised. AARP 2019; July 1.
    https://www.aarp.org/health/conditions-treatments/info-2019/pneumonia-vaccine
    -recommendation.html.

41 Australian Technical Advisory Group on Immunisation (ATAGI). Australian Im-
    munisation Handbook, Australian Government Department of Health, Canberra,
    2018. https://immunisationhandbook.health.gov.au/vaccine-preventable-diseases
    /pneumococcal-disease.

42 Pneumovax 23 package insert. Merck. https://www.merck.com/product/usa/pi_circulars
    /p/pneumovax_23/pneumovax_pi.pdf.

43 Ibid.

44 Prevnar 13 package insert. Pfizer. https://www.fda.gov/files/vaccines%2C%20blood%20
    -%26%20biologics/published/Package-Insert—Prevnar-13.pdf.

45 Pneumokokvaccination har ført til færre alvorlige infektioner hos både vaccinerede og
    uvaccinerede. 2017; Oct. 12. https://www.ssi.dk/aktuelt/nyheder/2017/2017-10-epinyt
    -41-pneumok.

46 Anbefaling om indførelse af pneumokokvaccination i det danske børne-vaccinationspro-
    gram. *Sundhedsstyrelsen* 2007; June 25.

47 Gøtzsche PC. *Survival in an overmedicated world: look up the evidence yourself.*

48 WHO. Hepatitis B. 2018; Jan. 24. https://www.who.int/immunization/diseases
    /hepatitisB/en/.

49 WHO. Varicella vaccines position paper. 2014; June 20. https://www.who.int
    /immunization/policy/position_papers/varicella/en/.

50 Ibid.

CHAPTER 9

[1] Smallpox. https://en.wikipedia.org/wiki/Smallpox.

[2] Kringelbach L. Den sidste patient. *Information* 2000; Oct. 9.

[3] Smallpox. https://en.wikipedia.org/wiki/Smallpox.

[4] Kringelbach L. Den sidste patient.

[5] Gøtzsche PC. *Survival in an overmedicated world: look up the evidence yourself.* Copenhagen: People's Press; 2019.

[6] Gøtzsche PC. *Rational diagnosis and treatment. Evidence-based clinical decision-making,* 4th edition. Chichester: Wiley; 2007.

[7] Miller ER, Moro PL, Cano M, et al. Deaths following vaccination: What does the evidence show? *Vaccine* 2015;33:3288–92.

[8] Yellow fever. https://en.wikipedia.org/wiki/Yellow_fever.

[9] Miller ER, Moro PL, Cano M, et al. Deaths following vaccination: What does the evidence show?

[10] Ibid.

[11] Yellow fever.

[12] European Medicines Agency. Dengvaxia. 2018; Dec. 18. https://www.ema.europa.eu/en /medicines/human/EPAR/dengvaxia.

[13] Ibid.

[14] WHO. Questions and answers on dengue vaccines. 2018; Apr. 20. https://www.who .int/immunization/research/development/dengue_q_and_a/en/.

[15] Ibid.

[16] Dengvaxia controversy. https://en.wikipedia.org/wiki/Dengvaxia_controversy.

[17] Lema K, Blamont M. Philippines to charge officials of Sanofi, government over dengue vaccine. Reuters 2019; Mar. 3. https://www.reuters.com/article/us-sanofi-fr -philippines/philippines-to-charge-officials-of-sanofi-government-over-dengue-vaccine -idUSKCN1QI41L.

CHAPTER 10

[1] WHO. Ten threats to global health in 2019. www.who.int/emergencies/ten-threats-to -global-health-in-2019.

[2] Brewer NT, Chapman GB, Rothman AJ, et al. Increasing vaccination: putting psychological science into action. *Psychol Sci Public Interest* 2017;18:149–207.

[3] Gøtzsche PC. *Deadly medicines and organised crime: How big pharma has corrupted health care.* London: Radcliffe Publishing; 2013; Gøtzsche PC. *Deadly psychiatry and organised denial.* Copenhagen: People's Press; 2015.

[4] Ibid.

[5] Ibid.

[6] Skowronski DM, De Serres G, Crowcroft NS, et al. Association between the 2008–09 seasonal influenza vaccine and pandemic H1N1 illness during spring–summer 2009: four observational studies from Canada. *PLoS Med* 2010;7:e1000258.

[7] Gøtzsche PC. *Death of a whistleblower and Cochrane's moral collapse.* Copenhagen: People's Press; 2019.

Index